DIABETES-RELATED KNOWLEDGE

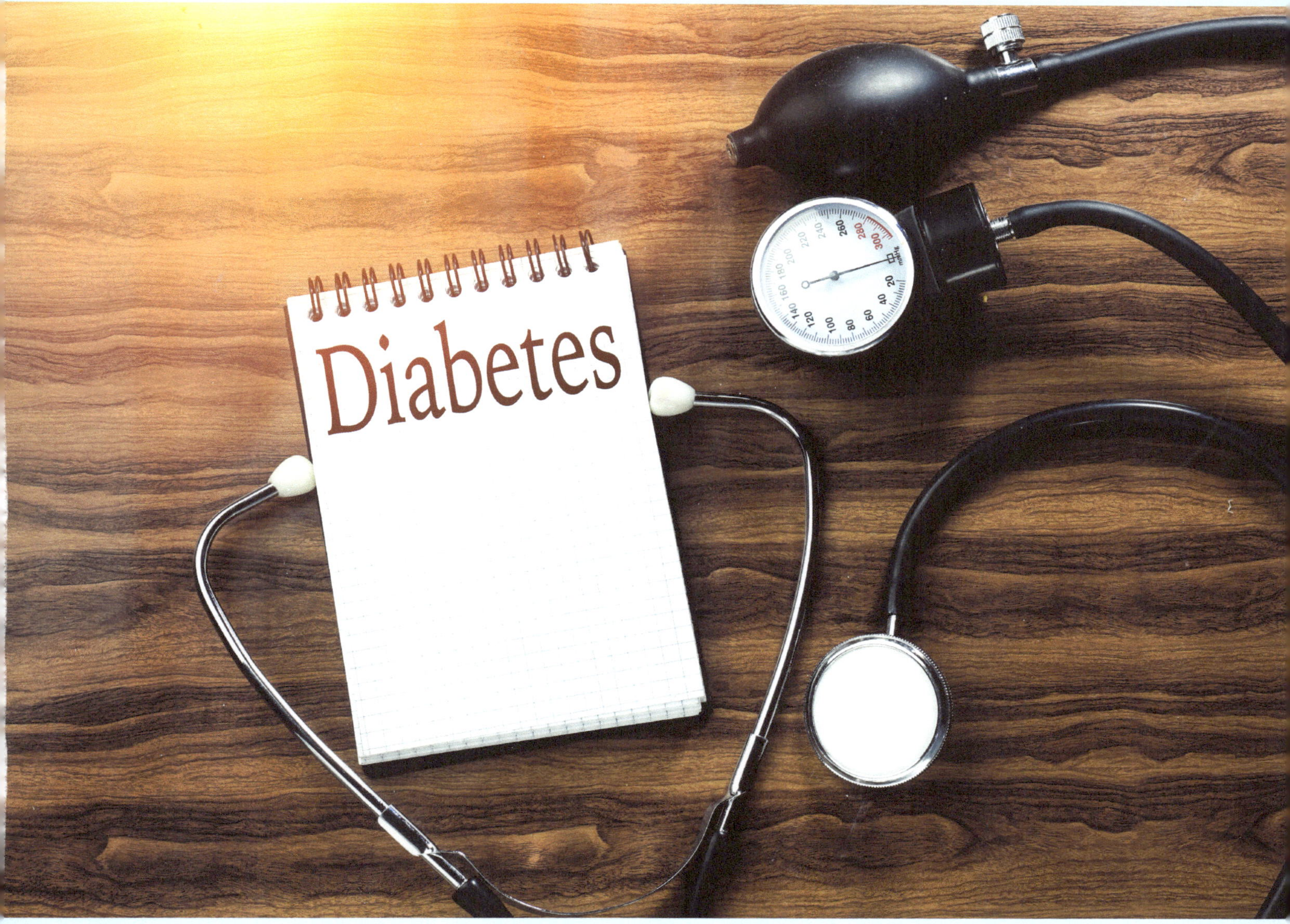

Diabetes

AMONG MIDDLE-AGED AFRICAN AMERICAN WOMEN IN NORTH TEXAS

DR. VICTOR AKHIDENOR

To order additional copies of this book, contact:
Xlibris
1-888-795-4274
www.Xlibris.com
Orders@Xlibris.com

ISBN: Softcover   978-1-7960-6219-9
         Hardcover   978-1-7960-6220-5
         EBook   978-1-7960-6218-2

Print information available on the last page

Rev. date: 10/09/2019

DIABETES-RELATED
KNOWLEDGE
AMONG MIDDLE-AGED
AFRICAN AMERICAN
WOMEN IN NORTH TEXAS

DR. VICTOR AKHIDENOR

A Dissertation Presented in Partial Fulfillment
Of the Requirements for the Degree of
Doctor of Health Administration

University of Phoenix

The Dissertation Committee for Victor Akhidenor certifies approval of the following dissertation:

EXPLORING DIABETES-RELATED KNOWLEDGE AMONG MIDDLE-AGED

BLACK/AFRICAN-AMERICAN WOMEN IN NORTH TEXAS

Committee:

Craig Follins, PhD, Chair

Darnell Anderson, PhD, Committee Member

Joann Kovacich, PhD, Committee Member

Craig Follins

_____

Craig Follins

Darnell Anderson

_____

Darnell Anderson

Joann Kovacich

_____

Joann Kovacich

K. Eye

_____

Hinrich Eylers, PhD
Vice Provost, Doctoral Studies
University of Phoenix

Date Approved: 12/10/2018 _____

Table of Contents

ABSTRACT _____ 1

DEDICATION _____ 3

ACKNOWLEDGEMENTS _____ 5

CHAPTER 1: Introduction _____ 7

Background of the Problem _____ 8

Statement of the Problem _____ 10

Purpose of the Study _____ 11

Significance of the Problem _____ 12

Nature of the Study _____ 14

Research Questions and Hypothesis _____ 15

Operational Definition of Variables _____ 16

The Conceptual Framework _____ 16

Definition of Terms _____ 20

Assumptions _____ 21

Scope of the Study _____ 21

Limitations Delimitations _____ 21

Summary _____ 22

CHAPTER 2: Literature Review _____ 23

Literature Search Strategy _____ 23

Theoretical Foundation _____ 24

Historical Overview _____ 29

Empirical Research on Key Variables and/or Constructs Self-care Management _____ 30

Diabetes Self-management Education _____ 44

Gaps in the Literature _____ 44

Conclusion _____ 45

Summary _____ 46

CHAPTER 3: Methodology _____ 47

Research Approach Appropriateness _____ 47

Research Design Appropriateness _____ 48

Population and Sampling Frame _____ 49

Inclusion Criteria _____ 50

Informed Consent _____ 51

Confidentiality _____ 52

Geographic Location _____ 52

Operational Definition of Variables and/or Constructs _____ 52

Data Collection _____ 53

Data Storage and Preparation. _____ 54

Instrumentation _____ 55

Demographic Questionnaire _____ 55

Data Analysis _____ 58

Validity and Reliability_____ 61

Summary _____ 63

CHAPTER 4: Results _____ 65

Research Design and Methods _____ 65

Research Questions and Hypothesis _____ 65

Population and Sampling _____ 66

Data Collection _____ 66

Self-care Knowledge _____ 70

Self-care Management _____ 73

Self-care Efficacy _____ 78

Data Analysis _____ 81

Summary _____ 82

CHAPTER 5: Conclusion and Recommendations_____ 85

Summary of the Findings _____ 85

Findings and Interpretation_____ 86

Strengths and Limitations _____ 88

Recommendations _____ 89

Summary _____ 90

Conclusions _____ 90

REFERENCES _____ 93

APPENDIX A: Advertising Flyer _____ 101

APPENDIX B: Letter of Informed Consent _____ 103

APPENDIX C: Demographic Questionnaire _____ 105

APPENDIX D: Diabetes Knowledge Test _____ 107

APPENDIX E: The Summary of Diabetes Self-Care Activities Scale _____ 111

APPENDIX F: Stanford Diabetes Self-care efficacy Scale ___ 115

APPENDIX G: Results of Binary Logistics Regression Model _____ 119

LIST OF TABLES

Table 1. Summary of the Literature reviewed by topic area. _____ 24

Table 2. Scoring the SDSCA scale _____ 56

Table 3. Cross-section of Studies that have used the SDSCA Scale _____ 56

Table 4. Cross-section of Studies that have used the Stanford Self-care efficacy scale _____ 57

Table 5. Statistical Approach to Data Analysis _____ 60

Table 6. Demographic Characteristics of the Participants_____ 67

Table 7. Descriptive statistics for Self-care Knowledge, Self-care Management and Self-care Efficacy _____ 68

Table 8. Bivariate Correlations between Diabetes Education, and Self-care Knowledge, Management, and Efficacy 69

Table 9. Descriptive Statistics of Self-care Knowledge _____ 71

Table 10. Descriptive Statistics of Self-care Management _____ 74

Table 11. Characteristics of Respondents Who Correctly Engaged in Self-care Behaviors_____ 74

Table 12. Correlations of Self-care management and Demographic variables_____ 76

Table 13. Correlations of Self-care knowledge and Self-care management behaviors _____ 77

Table 14. Descriptive Statistics of Self-care Efficacy _____ 78

Table 15. Characteristics of Participants with High Self-care Efficacy Score _____ 79

Table 16. Correlations of Self-care efficacy and Demographic variables_____ 79

Table 17. Contribution of variables to the model_____119

LIST OF FIGURES

Figure 1. The Health Belief Model (Becker & Rosenstock, 1984) _____ 17

Figure 2. Modified Health Belief Model (Becker & Rosenstock, 1984). _____ 19

Figure 3. Diabetes as a Risk Factor for Certain Cancer Types (RR[95%CI]). (Yeh et al., 2015). _____ 40

Figure 4. Plot of G*power for sample size selection (Faul et al., 2009) _____ 50

Figure 5. Histogram of Self-care Knowledge Scores _____ 73

Figure 6. Histogram of Self-care management scores _____ 77

Figure 7. Distribution of the Self-care Efficacy Scale _____ 80

ABSTRACT

This was a descriptive, quantitative correlational study examining the relationships between self-care knowledge, self-care management, and self-care efficacy in middle-aged Black/African American women with type II diabetes in north Texas. Prior research had indicated that Black/African American women are disproportionately affected by diabetes and have a higher incidence of diabetesrelated complications including: lower extremity amputation, end-stage renal disease, death from cardiovascular complications, and re-hospitalizations. Over 20 million Americans in the U.S. have diagnosed diabetes and the prevalence of the disease particularly among Black/African Americans is alarming. Texas ranks 10th in the nation for people with diabetes. Obesity, which is a major risk factor for type II diabetes has seen an increase in Texas from 10.7% in 1990 to over 33% in 2017. Unarguably, these disparities disproportionately affect Black/African American women as more adult women are denied access to affordable quality healthcare services and Medicaid insurance. One hundred twenty respondents completed an online Likert-type survey hosted on SurveyMonkey. Data was representative from demographics groups at churches, clinics, and public libraries. The relationships between self-care efficacy and selfcare knowledge, self-care efficacy and self-care management, and self-care knowledge and self-care management were tested. Results indicated a moderate correlation but statistically significant relationship among the variables. A binary logistic regression model found diabetes education significantly predicted selfcare maintenance. More research is needed before developing a culturally based targeted education program aimed at improving healthcare knowledge and maintenance among high risk individuals.

DEDICATION

This dissertation is dedicated to God, and to my late mother Christina Ehanlen Abhulimen who passed to glory on May 5, 1985. She inspired me to go to school though she was not educated. We toiled in the farmland to raise money for school fees and related expenses. She also taught me to work hard to achieve what I wanted in life without depending on human beings who may fail you at time of need. I am deeply indebted to my family who supported me with cash and words of encouragement during this arduous journey to success. I am grateful to God that a journey I started with so many uncertainties has come to an end.

Whenever I felt like throwing in the towel a few times due to challenges of life events, the encouragement of friends and families gave me the spirit of endurance and the motivation to keep hope alive. I must say a big thank you to my classmate and friend Dr. Allieu M. Shaw who encouraged me not to give up when I was frustrated and felt like quitting. It would not have been easy to thread on this road to success, but keeping positive people in my life made it possible. I am especially grateful and thankful to my lovely wife Precious Akhidenor and children Chris Akhidenor, Trinity Akhidenor, Edewede Akhidenor, and Ebehireme Akhidenor who always teased me of being in school at my old age. I say to them "education is an invaluable tool to have regardless of age". A big thanks to my cousin Ebanehita Okosun whose contribution to my success is immensely appreciated. God bless my friends and family.

ACKNOWLEDGEMENTS

I gratefully acknowledge the contributions of my dissertation committee through their support, feedbacks, and encouragement during the dissertation process. My committee chair Dr. Craig Follins highly motivated me and contributed to my success. I could not have done it without his resilient effort to make sure I am on the right track. I also acknowledge my methodologist Dr. Bob Amason whose feedbacks were invaluable.

My sincere appreciation to all those who participated in my survey and to the organizations that made it possible. Many thanks to my peers who helped critic my survey instruments and offered feedbacks in return. My appreciation to Dr. Joann Kovacich and Dr. Darnell Anderson for their patient and immense contribution. My sincere gratitude and appreciation to my best friend and mentor Dr. Allieu M. Shaw who contributed immensely to the success of my dissertation process. Thank you for all your feedback and contribution.

The encouragement and support from my friends, co-workers and wellwishers during this journey will never be forgotten. I owe my dissertation chair Dr. Craig Follins a tremendous debt of gratitude for his compassion and encouragement since he accepted to head my committee. God bless each and every one for their respective contributions to this dissertation process. God blessing!

CHAPTER 1

Introduction

Diabetes is a progressive chronic disease that is affecting millions of middle-aged Black/African American women in the United States and hundreds of millions worldwide. It is a metabolic condition that does not adequately process carbohydrates for energy, resulting in high levels of glucose in the bloodstream. Type-2 diabetes (T2DM) accounts for roughly 90% of all cases of diabetes. People with diabetes suffer a higher burden of psychosocial and psychological disorder (Chew, Shariff-Ghazali, & Fernandez, 2014).

Middle-aged Black/African American women are 1.9 times more likely to be diagnosed with diabetes, are 2.3 times more likely to be diagnosed with endstage renal disease, are 2.4 times more likely to die from diabetes-related complications, are 1.7 times more likely to be hospitalized from diabetes-related complications, and are twice as likely to have lower extremity amputation compared to their non-Hispanic white counterparts (Health and Human Services [HHS], 2015). This may be associated with a limited knowledge of the disease or the lack of capacity to actively engage in the self-care processes. In Texas, the prevalence of diagnosed diabetes in middle-aged Black/African Americans (45 to 64 years of age) is 16.2%. Texas ranks 10th in the nation for people diagnosed with diabetes and based on epidemiological data, diabetes is the 6th leading cause of death in the state (CHS, 2012). Chapter 1 discusses the background and purpose of the study, the theoretical framework used to guide the study, definition of terms, assumptions, scope, limitations, research questions and hypotheses, and implications for leadership.

Background of the Problem

Diabetes is increasing in prevalence in the U.S, particularly among middle-aged Black/African-Americans. Roughly 9.5% or 29.1 million people aged 20 years and older in the U.S. have diabetes including 8.1 million people with undiagnosed diabetes. Based on data from the National Health Interview Survey (NHIS), the prevalence of diagnosed diabetes among adults in the U.S. increased from 5.1% in 1997 to an estimated 30.3 million (9.4%) in 2015. In 2015, an estimated 10.7 million middle-aged adult Americans had diagnosed diabetes and an additional 3.6 million had prediabetes. Among middle-aged adults, 11.7 million women had diagnosed diabetes compared to 11.3 million men. In a 2007-2009 NHIS, 1,052,000 (13.7%) new cases of diagnosed diabetes among middle-aged adult Americans (45 – 64 years) were recorded (CDC, 2015a). Nationally, the prevalence of diabetes in Black/African-Americans is 12.7% in 2015. Roughly 1.5 million adult Americans are diagnosed with diabetes each year (ADA, 2018).

In Texas, the prevalence of diabetes is on the rise. According to the NHIS, the prevalence of diabetes in Texas rose from 10.2% in 2011 to 11.5% in 2015. The CDC estimates that roughly one in three Americans born after 2000 may develop diabetes during their lifetime. Diabetes is reported to be the 7th leading cause of death in the U.S. Texas ranks as the 2nd largest state in the U.S. with a population estimate of 27.8 million people. African-Americans represent 12.6% of the population compared to 39.1% of Hispanics or Latinos and 42.6% of nonHispanic whites (Census, 2017). The prevalence of diabetes among African-Americans is 17% in 2015.

A 2013 Texas Behavioral Risk Factor Survey showed a high prevalence of diabetes among African-Americans (13.3%) compared to non-Hispanic Whites (10.3%) and other cultures. Evidence from research show non-white patients have higher HbA1c levels and hospitalizations per year compared with non-Hispanic white patients (Rothman et al., 2008; Egede & Gogo-Jack, 2005; Mayer-Davis et al., 2009; American Diabetes Association [ADA], 2012). Multiple studies have asserted in the literature of a high risk of decreased psychological well-being among patients with diabetes (Chew, Shariff-Ghazali, & Fernandez, 2014).

Diabetes is a complex disease with multiple severe co-morbidities. Diabetes is characterized as the leading cause of blindness and end-stage renal disease (Konen, Summerson, Bell, & Curtis, 1999; CDC, 2012), non-traumatic lower limb amputations (Harris, 2006; CDC, 2012); heart disease and stroke, and is the seventh leading cause of death in the U.S (NIH, 2012; CDC, 2012). The risk for developing diabetes increases with age (Mooradian, McLaughlin, Boyer, & Winter, 1999), race/ethnicity, the environment, and genetic factors. Selvin (2006) found middle-aged adults with diabetes had different set of co-morbidities and poor glycemic control compared with 42% of adults that were diagnosed later in life.

In 2012, an estimated 892,000 (12 per 1,000) new cases of diabetes was diagnosed among middle-aged adults compared to 371,000 (3.6 per 1,000) new cases among adults aged 20 to 44 years (ADA, 2017). African-American women are particularly vulnerable to major complications associated with the disease, in part because of the lack of self-care efficacy in self-care behaviors (Mayer-Davis, Beyer, Bell,

Dabella, D'Agostino, Imperatore, Lawrence, & Rodriguez, 2009). Despite the similarities in intervention and self-care education programs, African Americans lack the knowledge, skills and the self-care efficacy to maintain tighter glycemic control compared to their non-Hispanic Whites. Earlier studies have demonstrated that Black/African-Americans relatively have higher self-esteem (Hughes & Demo, 1989) but recent studies show Black/African Americans have a general awareness of the disease but there are conceptual gaps in knowledge about susceptibility and the risk factors (Ballis-Berry et al. 2015).

The projected case of diabetes in Texas is estimated to reach 2.9 million people by 2030. In a 2013 BRFSS survey, 15.8% of middle-aged adults have diabetes compared to 1.6% of adults aged 18 – 29 years old, and 5.1% of adults aged 30 – 44 years old. Among the 2013 BRFSS survey of diagnosed adults with diabetes, 10.4% are females, 13.7% are middle-aged, and the highest prevalence of diagnosed diabetes was found in African-Americans (13.3%) compared to 10.3% of non-Hispanic Whites, and 11.9% of Hispanics. The four counties in Texas with the highest prevalence of diagnosed diabetes are Bexar County, Dallas County, Harris County, and Tarrant County (Texas Department of State Health Services [Texas DHS], 2013).

Diabetes is listed among the top ten leading causes of death in Texas. The mortality rate for middle-aged Black/African-American women with diabetes as the primary cause of death is disproportionately higher in Texas than their nonHispanic White counterparts. African-Americans were 2.5 times more likely to die from the disease compared with their non-Hispanic white counterparts (ADA, 2007). In a 2015 annual survey, the age-adjusted annual mortality rate from diabetes as a primary cause of death in Texas was 82.6 deaths compared with 67.6 deaths per 100,000 nationally for all demographics. Among Texas demographics, the diabetes-related death rate was significantly lower for females (68.0 per 100,000) compared to males (101.0 deaths per 100,000). The *Healthy People 2020* (HP2020) goal is to reduce diabetes-related deaths from the baseline of 74.0 deaths per 100,000 in 2007 to 66.6 deaths per 100,000. However, African Americans disproportionately died at a rate of 123.8 deaths compared to 80.3 deaths per 100,000 for non-Hispanic whites (U.S. Health and Human Services [HHS], 2017). In Dallas County, middle-aged Black/African-American women disproportionately died at a rate of 48.5 deaths per 100,000 compared with 21.8 deaths per 100,000 for their non-Hispanic white counterparts (CDC/Wonder, 2015).

Statement of the Problem

The general problem is, Black/African Americans are twice as likely to have lower extremity amputation compared to their non-Hispanic white counterparts, are 2.3 times more likely to be diagnosed with end-stage renal disease, are 2.4 times more likely to die from diabetes-related complications, and are 1.7 times more likely to be hospitalized from diabetes-related complications (Health and Human Services [HHS], 2015). Weinger (2007) asserted that people who exhibit low levels of self-care efficacy were less likely to engage in effective treatment protocols and self-care in attaining strong glycemic control, and are therefore more likely to suffer from diabetes complications.

The specific problem is, middle-aged Black/African American Women with T2DM have less self-care knowledge and low self-care efficacy to engage in self-care management of diabetes and its related-complications (Al Aboudi et al., 2017). According to Chen et al. (2014), the lack of disease-specific self-care knowledge may contribute to low self-care efficacy and the individual's ability to perform self-care management. A quantitative, descriptive study with a correlation design was performed to assess the relationship between the individuals' level of self-care efficacy, their knowledge of diabetes, and their ability to perform self-care management in middle-aged Black/African-American women with T2DM in north Texas.

Research is needed to determine whether pharmacologic treatment protocols are sufficient to increase self-care efficacy and promote self-care knowledge and self-care management in middle-aged Black/African-American women with T2DM. According to Cheng et al. (2012), markers of Socioeconomic Status (income, education, occupation) and BMI explain only 30% of the variability in glycated hemoglobin (HbA1c) levels observed in Black/AfricanAmericans, suggesting that behavioral influences, genetic factors, and nonpharmacologic factors may explain some of the variance in disease risk. However, Black/African-Americans, despite the pharmacologic interventions, have a 0.85% higher than average HbA1c scores, negative medication beliefs, and lower selfcare efficacy compared to their non-Hispanic white counterparts (CDC, 2013; Spruill et al., 2013).

Low socioeconomic status is an impediment in the delivery of equitable care. A review of socioeconomic disparities in the United States across multiple health indicators (diabetes, heart disease, obesity) and socioeconomic groups found people in low socioeconomic status and who were least educated were more likely to consistently exhibit health deficits (Braveman, Cubbin, Egerter, Williams, & Pamuk, 2010). However, evidence suggests that middle-aged Black/African-American women with Type II diabetes exhibit poor self-care skills and adverse complications even after controlling for SES differences. In spite of the disparities in SES, ineffective self-care skills or poor glycemic control may be influenced by psychosocial and behavioral factors which are known to impede sustainable behavior changes in people with diabetes (Weinger, 2007).

Researchers who have examined the effects of psychosocial stressors on self-care behaviors in people with diabetes has had mixed results. One study examined the relationship between stress and glucose regulation among people with diabetes but the findings were mixed (Lloyd, Mathews, Wing, & Orchard, 1992). Al-Khawaldeh, Al-Hassan, and Froelicher (2012) examined the relationship between diabetes self-care efficacy and diabetes self-care behaviors and glycemic control, and posited that behavioral counseling is critical to building confidence in managing diabetes.

A similar study was conducted in Britain to determine the impediments to diabetes management among British subjects. The study was a mixed method study involving 118 participants of which 91.5% were white British subjects, 93 (78.8%) had Type II diabetes, 54(45.8%) were females, and 49 (21.2%) were between the ages 46 and 65 years. Researchers found 40.2% of the participants did not know their HbA1c indicating that the participants lack knowledge of selfcare. According to the American Diabetes Association, the lack of attaining desirable (HbA1c ≤ 7.0) including lowering blood pressure and LDL cholesterol could increase the risk of diabetes complications (Elliott, Harris, & Laird, 2016). The effects of psychosocial stressors on poor behavioral outcomes in self-care management is not well understood (Kordas, Ardoino, Ciccariello, Manay, Ettimger, Cook, & Queirolo, 2011). The interest to explore the relationship between knowledge, efficacy, and self-care stems from the observation that psychosocial stressors and social stressors (discrimination, poverty, social anxiety, social inequality, and unscheduled life events) are often spatially correlated, and that either of these factors may inhibit the efficacy of the individual to engage in effective self-care behaviors.

Purpose of the Study

The purpose of this descriptive, quantitative, correlational study was to assess the association and magnitude of the relationship, if any, between self-care knowledge, self-care efficacy, and self-care management in middle-aged Black/African-American women (45 – 64 years of age) with T2DM in Dallas or Tarrant County, north Texas. The variables to be explored in this study are selfcare efficacy, self-care knowledge, and self-care management. Self-care efficacy refers to "people's judgments about their capability to perform particular tasks. Task-related self-care efficacy increases the effort and persistence towards challenging tasks; therefore, increasing the likelihood that they will be completed" (Barling & Beattie, 1983, as cited in Axtell & Parker, 2003, p. 114). In this study, self-care efficacy was measured by the Stanford Diabetes Self-care efficacy Scale (Appendix F).

Knowledge is defined as "facts, information, and skills acquired through experience or education; the theoretical or practical understanding of a subject" ("Knowledge,"2017). Operationally, self-care knowledge refers to a patient's ability to acquire the information and skills through experience or education to facilitate performance of self-care. Self-care knowledge was measured by the Diabetes Knowledge Test (Appendix D).

Self-care management as defined within the context of this study is the process of "teaching individuals to manage their diabetes" (Norris et al., 2001, p. 561). Self-care management refers to a patient's ability to engage in the "daily activities that individuals undertake to keep their illness under control, minimize its impact on physical health status and functioning, and cope with the psychosocial sequelae of the illness" (Gallant, 2003, p. 170). Self-care management was measured by the Summary of Diabetes Self-care Activities Scale (Appendix E). Diabetes Self-management Education is the method of facilitating knowledge, skills, and the ability for appropriate self-management behavior in people with diabetes. The knowledge acquired in-turn helps patients improve clinical outcomes and self-management behavior to reduce the risk of secondary complications (Appendix C) (Funnell et al. (2010).

Descriptive research is appropriate for this study because the primary objective of this research is to determine "what is" to investigate the relationship between multiple variables (Glass & Hopkins, 1984). Descriptive research can include quantitative data and can be used to report correlation or association between variables. Descriptive research can be used to collect data and organize, tabulate, or describe the data collection. Descriptive research is unique in the sense that it can include multiple variables and unlike other research methods, it requires only a single variable (Borg & Gall, 1996). For instance, although descriptive research cannot be used to explain causation, however, it can be used to explain aspects of a phenomenon or the behavior of a sample population.

A quantitative approach is appropriate for this study because it involves testing the differences in relationships and examining the cause and effect connections between variables (LoBiondo-Wood & Harber, 2009). A correlational design is appropriate because it determines to what degree and direction a relationship exists between two or more variables. Although a correlation does not imply causation between the variables; however, it specifies concomitant variations in the scores on the variables (Hauke & Kossowski, 2011).

Significance of the Problem

Significance for Research. The empirical nature of this study could contribute significantly to the existing body of knowledge by understanding human behavior and decision-making in health and illness. Behavioral and social science research helps to predict, prevent, and manage illness in individuals. This study explored human behaviors concerning perceptions of risk and decisionmaking with the heath regimen of people with T2DM. The outcome from this study could enhance knowledge about the phenomenon of adherence to a health regimen from a health and behavioral perspective. The findings from this study may further contribute to significant foundational information about the relationships among the constructs being investigated in middle-aged Black/African-American women with T2DM. Thus the outcomes could be significant and contribute to knowledge in behavioral research for Black/African-American women with T2DM.

Significance for Theory. The proposed framework is a frequently used theory that is relative to health behaviors and health decision-making. The significance of this study for theory is that the empirical nature of this research can help to visualize the relationships between the constructs being measured and its impact on behavior. Since the model uses psychological constructs to predict health behaviors the findings could be used to explain why patients avoid or delay preventative measures, why people react to perceptions of a threat of acquiring a disease, or why people are not compliant with medical regimens even in the face of a perceived threat of the severity of the illness. The significance of this study to the HBM is that the findings from empirical data could be further used to modify the constructs to expand the theory.

Significance for Practice. Findings from this study may hold significance to the nursing practice whose role in proving knowledge and quality care has evolved over the past decade in response to the shifting demands and expectations of people with diabetes. The significance of the findings from this study may contribute new knowledge to the already existing body of knowledge in the nursing practice. For example, the findings can be used to determine the prevalence of diabetes among a target population, the strength of the association among the variables being explored, and to inform decision-making in nursing practice in order to improve healthcare-related activities. The knowledge obtained from this study may help to empower nurses/patients to make decisions in ways to improve their capabilities for self-care and hence meet the requirements for adherence to treatment regimen. Findings may further hold significance to healthcare practitioners who may try to understand a patient's state of mental health and design non-pharmacologic interventions to eliminate the risk of diabetes-related distress, depression, preventable hospitalizations, and reduced mortality.

Significance for Leadership. The proposed study may be vital to health care leaders that have a vested interest in improving the health of their communities and constituents. This study may also be vital to local governments that create policies that affect the health of their constituents. Findings from the study may hold significance to healthcare leaders in particular by: (a) using the results of the research to improve program effectiveness to make better decisions in allocating resources, (b) developing policy strategy, drafting legislation, evaluating proposed legislation or monitoring program progress and effectiveness, (c) working with informed coalitions to bring together a diverse range of people, organizations, and educators to broaden their scope and perspective in understanding the issues prior to developing policy, (d) making "informed policy decisions to improve the effectiveness of state public health programs and improve the health of the population" (Council of State Governments, 2008, p.iii).

Nature of the Study

Overview of Research Approach. The proposed study was designed as a correlational study to determine whether there was a relationship between selfcare efficacy, self-care knowledge and self-care management in middle-aged Black/African-American women with T2DM. Several studies have addressed behavioral influences for people with diabetes. However, there is paucity in empirical research about behavioral influences on self-care in middle-aged Back/African-American women with T2DM. The quantitative approach was appropriate for this study for several reasons – (a) it is rooted in the post-positivist paradigm which enables the researcher to determine how different causes interact and/or influence outcomes, (b) it tests the differences in relationships between variables (LoBionodo-Wood & Harber, 2009), (c) it enables the researcher to quantify the relationship between and among the variables, (d) it allows for the development and answer to test theories or hypothesis, (e) it assumes the sample is a representative of the population, and (f) it primarily uses deductive reasoning to establish a theoretical framework in which the concepts have already been reduced to variables, and then develop evidence to test, or assess whether the framework or theory is supported (Burns & Grove, 2005). The qualitative method did not seem appropriate because qualitative designs are rooted in the naturalistic paradigm and the objective of this study was not to examine human experiences in natural settings or use textual data to analyze the experiences being studied (Burns & Grove, 2005).

Overview of Research Design. A correlational design was appropriate for the proposed study because it will enable to determine the degree and the direction of the relationship between and within the variables self-care efficacy, self-care knowledge, and self-care management. Correlational design was a way of systematically investigating the nature of relationships or associations between and among variables. Shapiro (2011) postulated that although correlation determines the degree and direction of a relationship among the variables; however, its limitations is that "it does not provide any information about the magnitude—or the size—of the relationship between variables" (p. 3).

By employing a quantitative approach using a self-reported survey, it was possible to collect data from a large audience and to make generalizations from the survey sample to a wider population. The data collected from the survey are usually quantitative in nature and can be analyzed using descriptive and inferential statistics. The knowledge generated from the survey was predominantly descriptive or explanatory.

Self-reported surveys have the advantages of being: (a) a cost effective way to collect data, (b) administered remotely using a variety of communications platforms, (c) validity, reliability, and statistical significance can be determined, (d) geographical dependence can be eliminated using a variety of communications platforms, (e) a broad range of data (such as attitudes, beliefs, behavior, values, and demographics) can be collected from a large audience within a limited time frame, and (f) multiple variables can be collected and analyzed. Three instruments and a demographic questionnaire were used to collect data for this proposed study. The survey instruments were all appropriate for the collection of quantitative data. A detail description of the instruments is discussed in Chapter 3 under "Instruments".

Research Questions and Hypothesis

The research question and the hypotheses in this study are as follows:

RQ# 1 – What is the relationship, if any, between self-care efficacy and self-care knowledge in middle-aged Black/African-American women with T2DM in north Texas?

$H1_0$ – There is no statistically significant relationship between self-care efficacy and self-care knowledge in middle-aged Black/African-American women with T2DM in north Texas.

$H1_1$ – There is a statistically significant relationship between self-care efficacy and self-care knowledge in middle-aged Black/African-American women with T2DM in north Texas.

RQ# 2 – What is the relationship, if any, between self-care efficacy and self-care management in middle-aged Black/African-American women with T2DM in north Texas?

$H2_0$ – There is no statistically significant relationship between self-care efficacy and self-care management in middle-aged Black/African-American women with T2DM in north Texas.

$H2_1$ – There is a statistically significant relationship between self-care efficacy and self-care management in middle-aged Black/African-American women with T2DM in north Texas.

RQ# 3 – What is the relationship, if any, between self-care knowledge and self-care management in middle-aged Black/African-American women with T2DM in north Texas?

$H3_0$ – There is no statistically significant relationship between self-care knowledge and self-care management in middle-aged Black/African-American women with T2DM in north Texas.

$H3_1$ – There is a statistically significant relationship between self-care knowledge and self-care management in middle-aged Black/African-American women with T2DM in north Texas.

Operational Definition of Variables

The variables to be explored in this study were self-care efficacy, self-care knowledge, and self-care management. Self-care efficacy is the belief that an individual has the ability to create change by personal actions (Bandura, 1977). Operationally, *self-care efficacy* is determined by an individual's level of confidence to engage in diabetes management activities, such as blood glucose monitoring, engaging in diet and exercise, insulin administration, adhering to medication regimen, and responding to health challenges that may occur from time to time. This variable was measured on a categorical scale.

Self-care knowledge is the "facts, information, and skills acquired through experience or education; the theoretical or practical understanding of a subject" ("Knowledge,"2017). Operationally, self-care knowledge is a reasoned and reflective process. It refers to a patient's ability to acquire and use the information and skills through experience or education to facilitate performance of self-care. This variable was measured on a categorical scale.

Self-care management refers to a patient's ability to engage in the "daily activities that individuals undertake to keep their illness under control, minimize its impact on physical health status and functioning, and cope with the psychosocial sequelae of the illness" (Gallant, 2003, p. 170). Operationally, selfcare management in this context refers to "those activities individuals undertake in promoting their own health, preventing their own disease, limiting their own illness, and restoring their own health" (Levin, 1983, p.1). This variable was measured on a categorical scale. The three variables to be measured are discussed in Chapter 2 under "Empirical Search on Variables".

The Conceptual Framework

The Health Belief Model (HBM) was the conceptual framework (Figure 1.0) used as a guide for this study (Becker, 1974). The HBM was developed in the 1950s by social psychologist Hochbaum, Rosenstock, and Kegels working in the U.S. Public Health Services. The framework was developed in response to the failure of free tuberculosis (TB) health screening program, and a willingness to participate in preventive health behaviors such as immunizations and screening for diseases like diabetes, hypertension and cancer.

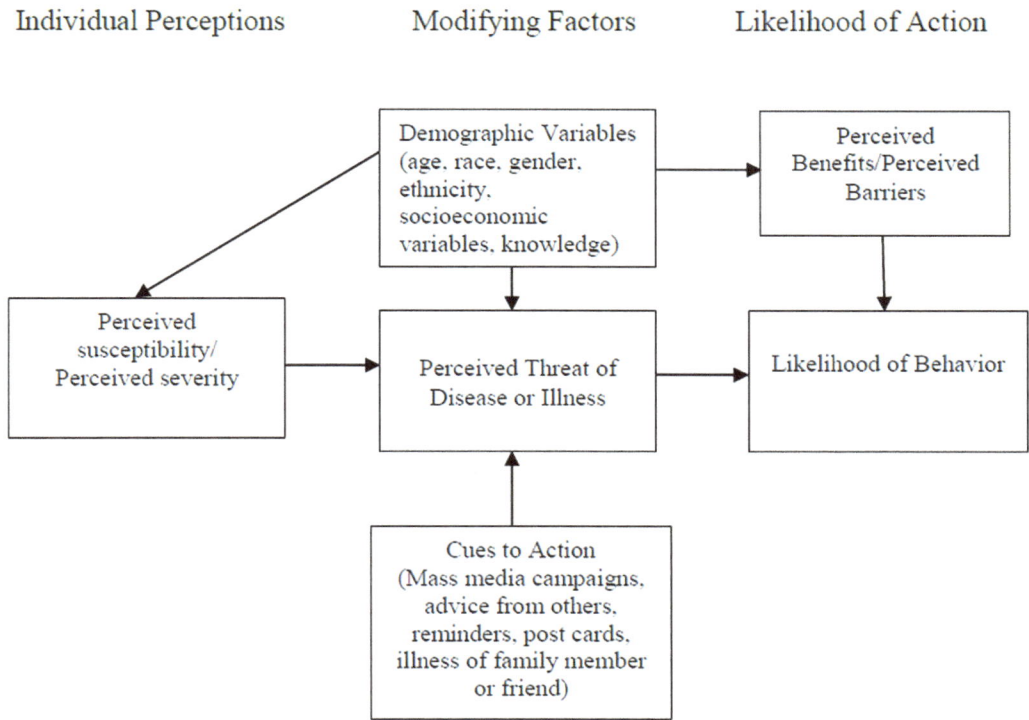

Figure 1. The Health Belief Model (Becker & Rosenstock, 1984)

The framework is used to understand health behavior or possible reasons for non-compliance with recommended health behavior (Becker & Rosenstock, 1984). Since the development of the model, it has been adapted to explore a variety of long- and short-term health behaviors, including sexual risk behaviors and the transmission of HIV/AIDS. According to Wallston and Wallston (1984), the HBM is the most frequently cited and applied psychosocial model used in behavioral research.

The HBM is a psychological model that attempts to explain and predict health behaviors. The model proposes that a person is more likely to take action in response to a perceived threat if the perceived benefits of the action outweigh the perceived barriers or costs of the health behavior (Rosenstock, 1974). In essence, even if an action is perceived to be beneficial, a person may decide not to take action to reduce a threat to their health if it is perceived as costly, painful, unpleasant or inconvenient. The HBM focuses on the attitudes and beliefs of individuals.

The HBM was selected because of its usefulness in explaining and predicting acceptance of health and medical care recommendations in a variety of health settings and health situations. The HBM model is grounded in six basic component: (a) perceived susceptibility (the degree to which an individual feels at risk of contracting a disease), (b) perceived severity (the degree of threat the disease imposes and its consequences), (c) perceived benefit (a person's belief in the efficacy of engaging in a particular behavior to reduce risk or seriousness of impact), (d) perceived barriers (a person's opinion of the tangible and intangible costs of engaging in a particular behavior to reduce risk or seriousness of impact), (e) cues to action (one's ability to trigger the decision-making process based on disease symptoms or mass media campaigns), and (f) self-care efficacy (confidence in one's ability to take action to reduce risk or seriousness of impact) (Rosenstock, 1974). More recently, other constructs such as cues to action, motivating factors, and self-care efficacy have been added to the HBM. The concept of self-care efficacy, or one's confidence in his or her ability to perform an action was added by Rosenstock and others in 1988 to help the model fit the challenges of changing unhealthy behaviors, such as living a sedentary life style, engaging in eating disorders or smoking.

As shown in Figure 1. the HBM is divided into three components: modifying factors, individual perceptions, and likelihood of action. Modifying factors such as self-care knowledge, self-care management, and self-care efficacy are variables that could indirectly influence individual behavior (Rosenstock, 1974). Individual perceptions are motives and thought processes that determine an individual's perception of their environment (Maiman & Becker, 1974). Likelihood of action encompasses an internal or external stimulus to trigger an individual to engage in an appropriate health behavior (Maiman & Becker, 1974) if the individual believes:

a) He or she is susceptible to contracting a disease

b) contracting the disease could pose adverse or severe consequences

c) taking action would reduce the burden of susceptibility to a disease

d) taking action would not require overcoming many barriers

(Rosenstock, 1974).

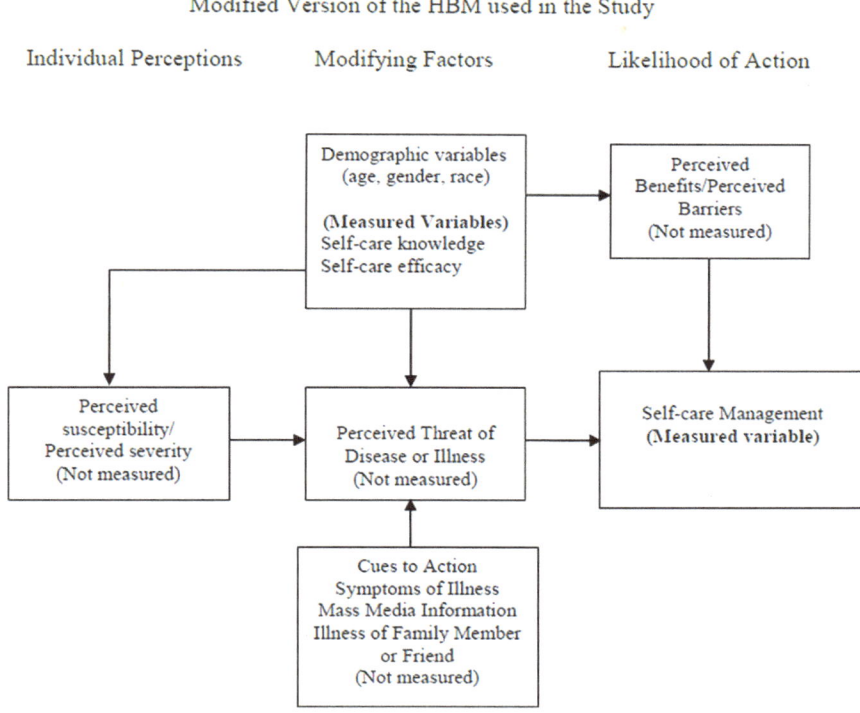

Figure 2. Modified Health Belief Model (Becker & Rosenstock, 1984).

The modified version of the HBM as used in this proposed study is shown in Figure 2. above. This study was to explore the strength and direction of the relationship between self-care efficacy, self-care knowledge, and self-care management in middle-aged Black/African-American women with T2DM in north Texas. Diabetes self-care management is a complex regimen of daily activties that includes diet, blood glucose testing, medication adherence, exercise, healthy coping skills, problem-solving skills, and risk-reduction behaviors (Shrivastava, Shrivastava, & Ramasamy, 2013). The implications of not adhereing to these regimens could potentially lead to adverse health outcomes including morbidity and mortality.

The focus of the HBM is on disease prevention and risk-reduction behavior. Accoridng to the modified HBM, individuals are more likely to engage in behaviors that will reduce a perceived threat of a disease or illness if he or she perceives the benefits would reduce their disease risk without substantial barriers such as costs, access to care, or knowledge of the disease. Research has shown that African-American women are disproportionately affected by the consequences of diabetes and are more susceptible to acquiring diabetes than their non-Hispanic white counterparts. The perception of susceptibility (or the risk of acquiring a disease such as diabetes) among African-American women and the perceived severity or seriousness of developing the consequences of the disease (such as neuropathy, nephropaty, retinopathy, cardiovascular disease, stroke, and lower peirpheral amputation) can trigger behavior change (such as adhering to medication regimen, improving diet and exercise) to avoid from acquiring the disease (Maddux & Rogers, 1998; Rosenstock, 1974).

Definition of Terms

The following definitions specify how variables are measured or assessed in a study. The variables listed here have operational use in this study.

Adherence – is the extent to which a person's behavior (making lifestyle changes, taking medications as prescribed, and following a recommended diet) corresponds with agreed upon recommendations from a health-care provider (WHO, 2003).

Diabetes Self-management Education is the method of facilitating knowledge, skills, and the ability for appropriate self-management behavior in people with diabetes. The knowledge acquired in-turn helps patients improve clinical outcomes and self-management behavior to reduce the risk of secondary complications (Funnell et al. (2010). Operationally, this variable is treated as a dichotomous variable.

Glycemic Control – refers to the level of glucose in the blood stream of people with diabetes. Glycemic control is synonymous with blood sugar control in which the body turns carbohydrates to be used for energy but the cells cannot use the glucose without the aid of insulin made by the pancreas (Bellenir & Dresser, 1995).

Hypoglycemia – is characterized as an abnormally low level of glucose in the blood stream. Symptoms marked by hypoglycemia include increased heart rate, confusion, sweating, dizziness, hunger and irritability (Tull & Roseman, 2005).

Hyperglycemia – is characterized as an abnormally high level of glucose in the blood stream. Symptoms marked by hyperglycemia include blurred vision, excess urination, rapid weight loss, polyuria and polydipsia (Tull & Roseman, 2005).

Polydipsia – is a medical condition linked to frequent urinary conditions and extreme thirst. These are known to be the first symptoms of diabetes (Bichet, Sterns, & Emmett, 2018).

Polyuria – is a medical condition similar to polydipsia – it involves frequent urination exceeding 3/L a day and causing extreme thirst (Bichet, Sterns, & Emmett, 2018).

Self-Care – is the "daily activities that individuals undertake to keep their illness under control, minimize its impact on physical health status and functioning, and cope with the psychosocial sequelae of the illness" (Gallant, 2003, p. 170). Self-care is synonymous with self-care behaviors.

Self-care Efficacy - is defined as "people's beliefs about their capabilities to produce designated levels of performance that exercise influence over events that affect their lives. Self-care efficacy beliefs determine "how people feel, think, motivate themselves and behave" (Bandura, 1994, p. 1). Self-care efficacy is derived from four major processes - cognitive, motivational, effective, and selection processes (Bandura, 1994).

Assumptions

Assumptions provide a basis to develop theories, hypothesis, and research instruments and, therefore, influence the development and implementation of research processes. The assumptions in this study were: (a) the participant's responses to the survey questions are honest, (b) not all of the participants in the sample may complete the study, (c) the sample size may be a true representation of the general population, and (d) the knowledge acquired from this study may be organized and distributed to the general population, (e) the sample subjects have sufficient computer literacy and cognition to respond to the online survey questions, (f) the respondents to the recruitment flyer are middle-aged, African American, women, have a medical diagnosis of T2DM, and true residents of north Texas.

Scope of the Study

The scope of a study defines its boundaries and population characteristics (Criswell, 2005). The scope of this study was limited to middle-aged Black/African-American women aged 45 to 64 years, with a diagnosis of T2DM and residing in north Texas. The instruments used to collect data from the participants for this study were the Demographic Questionnaire, the Diabetes Self-Care Activities Scale (SDSCA) (Toobert, Hampson, & Glasgow, 2000) to assess self-care behaviors, the Stanford Diabetes Self-care efficacy Scale to assess perceived self-care efficacy and the Michigan Diabetes Knowledge Test to assess self-care knowledge. The data was collected in an online environment using the SurveyMonkey® tool. The study used a convenience and snowball sampling method. Data for this study was collected until the sample size was attained. The approximate time allocated for data collection was 90 days from the date IRB approval was received. However, the response time was greater than was expected.

Limitations Delimitations

Limitations are restrictions of the study due to theoretical or methodological reasons, which may decrease the generalizability of the research findings. The limitations of this study were: (a) the sample size may not be sufficient to understand the significance between the independent and dependent variables, (b) the use of a convenience and snowball sampling methods may diminish the generalizability of the outcome of the study, (c) the cross-sectional nature of the study may not be used to determine causality between independent and dependent variables, (d) the validity and reliability of the study instruments are measured by their respective authors, (e) there was internal threats of sampling bias, selection bias, testing bias, instrument bias, self-report bias, and internal validity, (f) the study was limited to subjects that have access or link to the SurveyMonkey® platform via a computer, a smart phone, or a portable device. Participants were expected to self-report a medical diagnosis of T2DM. The instruments used in this study were written in English; thus, reading and understanding English was a requirement for participating in this study. This study was delimited to the design and methodology, sample, population, and data collected.

Summary

This chapter described the purpose of the study, the scope, assumptions, limitations, and delimitations, and the significance of the study. This study sought to determine whether there was a strong correlation between self-care knowledge, self-care efficacy and self-care management in middle-aged Black/African American women with T2DM. T2DM is one of the major leading causes of death in the U.S. It is a non-infections disease which has become a public health concern due to its prevalence, morbidity, and mortality rate. A health epidemiology survey by the Texas Department of Health shows that Black/African-Americans are disproportionately affected by the disease compared to their non-Hispanic white counterparts. The Health Belief Model (HBM) was used as the theoretical guide for this study. The HBM was selected because of its usefulness in explaining and predicting acceptance of health and medical care recommendations in a variety of health settings and health situations. Prospective participants were recruited using a convenience and snowball sampling method. Chapter 2 explored the epidemiology of diabetes in Texas. A review of the pertinent literature on the background of diabetes self-care behaviors among African-American women and the gaps that exist was discussed. Relevant studies dealing with non-pharmacologic psychosocial issues of diabetes self-care behaviors was used to compare and contrast with studies that have been published in the literature.

CHAPTER 2

Literature Review

The purpose of this descriptive, quantitative, correlational study was to assess the association and magnitude of the relationship, if any, between diabetesrelated knowledge, self-care efficacy, and self-care management in middle-aged Black/African-American women (45 – 64 years of age) with T2DM in north Texas. Chapter 1 discussed the purpose and rationale of the study, research questions and hypothesis, the scope, assumptions, limitations and delimitations, the significance of the study, and the conceptual framework that guided the study. Chapter 2 will discuss the literature on the relationship between self-care efficacy, self-care knowledge and self-care management and test the correlation between the variables.

Literature Search Strategy

The purpose of this literature review was to synthesize the published literature between 2011 and 2018, examining the relationship between perceived self-care efficacy and self-care knowledge and how it influences self-care behaviors in middle-aged Black/African-American women with T2DM. Title searches were conducted using the NIH libraries, CDC libraries, CINAHL, PubMed, Medline, PsycInfo, ProQuest, ERIC, EBSCOhost, Gale, and Cochrane databases. The searches were conducted using the following keywords: *diabetes, knowledge of self-care, self-care management, self-care behaviors, self-care efficacy, knowledge self-care efficacy, medication adherence, exercise self-care efficacy, diabetes quality of life, psychosocial constructs, diabetes-related distress, and depression.* Selection of literature was based on the relevance, applicability, currency, reliability, and validity of the literature to the proposed study.

In addition to using the search terms listed above, articles were selected based on meeting several criteria: what was known and written about the topic of interest (diabetes in middle-aged Black/African-American women), the central issues in the field of diabetes research (self-care behaviors, self-care efficacy, self-care knowledge, and diabetes education), the previous approaches to the topic of diabetes in Black/African-Americans, what other researchers have discovered in the field of diabetes research, and what is yet unknown in diabetes research. Table 1 presents a summary of the literature reviewed in support of the research study, its findings and presentations.

Table 1. Summary of the Literature reviewed by topic area.

Search Topics	Peer Reviewed Journals	Dissertations	Books	Others
Self-care knowledge	26	3	5	0
Self-care efficacy	18	1	1	0
Self-care Management	24	2	0	1
Self-care Behaviors	13	1	0	1
Self-care Education	9	3	0	1

Theoretical Foundation

The World Health Organization (WHO) characterized diabetes mellitus as a global epidemic with rising prevalence in low socioeconomic communities and since then has intensified its efforts to provide effective measures for the surveillance, prevention and control of the disease and its complications. The global prevalence of diabetes among adults 18 years and older has increased from 4.7% in 1980 to 8.5% in 2014. The number of persons with diabetes worldwide has risen from 108 million in 1980 to 422 million in 2014 and is expected to exceed 592 million people by 2035 to become the seventh leading cause of death worldwide (WHO, 2015; Guariguata, Whiting, Hambleton, Beagley, Linnenkamp, & Shaw, 2014).

Among the Organization for Economic Cooperation and Development (OECD) countries which includes the U.S, the prevalence of diabetes is expected to reach 108 million by 2030. According to the International Diabetes Federation (IDF, 2011), the U.S. ranks 6th among OECD countries for adults diagnosed with diabetes. In 2013, the U.S. ranked 8th among the countries with the highest rate of diabetes-related hospital readmissions (OECD, 2017). In spite of being the highest spender on healthcare among OECD countries, the U.S. ranks low in quality of care.

The greatest burden of diabetes – in prevalence, incidence, morbidity, and mortality is borne by non-Hispanic whites. The risk of acquiring diabetes is 80% higher in Black/African-Americans than their non-Hispanic white counterparts. The most common risk factors for T2DM are sedentary lifestyles, obesity, diet, high cholesterol and high blood pressure, age and family history of the disease (Fox et al., 2015). Roughly 4.9 million Black/African-Americans presently have diagnosed or undiagnosed diabetes.

Research also shows that Black/AfricanAmerican women have a disproportionate burden of diabetes and diabetes-related complications compared to their non-Hispanic white counterparts (CDC, 2016).

Managing diabetes requires knowledge of the disease and the efficacy to engage in a complex regimen of activities that includes clinical intervention and effective self-care practices such as diet, exercise, blood sugar testing, foot care, and medication adherence that are the cornerstones of diabetes self-care management. Diabetes is managed by means of pharmacologic and nonpharmacologic interventions. Pharmacological interventions are comprehensive medical care and patient education programs provided by clinicians to help patients maintain blood glucose levels within normal range in people with diabetes.

Patients are said to have "good" or "adequate" glycemic control if their preceding two- or three month average blood glucose levels (HbA1c < 7%). The HbA1c serves as a useful tool to determine if a patient has good glycaemic control. Patients with diabetes have an increased risk of developing cerebrovascular disease, peripheral vascular disease, and atherosclerotic cardiovascular disease. Adherence to tighter glycemic control to prevent future complications requires incorporating intensive lifestyle interventions such as smoking cessation, lowering systolic blood pressure to less than 130/80 mm HG, and reducing serum cholesterol to less than 150 mg/dl. Research shows that a one percent reduction in HbA1c can reduce the risk of macrovascular complications by 37%, the risk of myocardial infarction by 14% and diabetes-related deaths by 21% (Stratton et al., 2000).

Non-pharmacologic interventions are lifestyle changes incorporating physical exercise regimen and modification of nutrition intakes in the early or later stages of the onset of T2DM, combined with pharmacotherapy (Buysschaert & Hermans, 2004). Non-pharmacologic factors such as increased efficacy can be influenced by knowledge, lifestyle changes, social and cultural beliefs, and socioeconomic conditions which are equally important in the self-care process (Patel, Bhattacharya, & Butte, 2010). However, there is a scant of empirical evidence in the literature on non-pharmacologic factors that influence attitudes in the self-care process in middle-aged Black/African-American women with T2DM. The efficacy of non-pharmacologic interventions in the self-care process in Black/African-American women with T2DM has not been fully explored.

Research indicates that non-pharmacologic factors have had little or no attention in some settings. However, there is a general assertion among researchers that non-pharmacologic interventions are equally or more important compared to pharmacologic interventions for effective glycemic control (Mohebi et al., 2013). The social and emotional impact of managing diabetes and the high demands of diabetes-related therapy can contribute significantly to psychosocial deficits or low self-care efficacy in patients and their families thereby leading to poor glycemic control and adverse health outcomes (Expert Committee on the Diagnosis and Classification of Diabetes Mellitus, 2003).

Pousinho, Morgado, Falcao, and Alves (2016) found in a systematic review of 36 studies involving 5,761 participants that roughly 50% of people with diabetes are non-adherent to pharmacotherapy or lifestyle changes. The factors for non-adherence ranged from lack of economic resources, poor patient-provider communications, socio-cultural beliefs, inadequate insurance, medication side effects, complex treatment regimens, and psychosocial stressors to cognitive impairments. The World Health Organization (WHO) outlines five interacting dimensions affecting medication adherence: health system-related factors, patientrelated factors, therapy-related factors, socioeconomic-related factors, and condition-related factors (WHO, 2003).

Generally, psychosocial stressors in people with diabetes are widely explored and reported in the literature. In spite of its efficacy in the chronic disease process, the degree to which the findings generalize to middle-age Black/African-American female populations remain unclear. Research shows that African-Americans encounter higher levels of stress in several domains of socioeconomic disparities (National Research Council (US) Panel on Race, Ethnicity, and Health in Later Life, 2004). Psychosocial stressors are life influencing events that can cause distress in individuals, thereby, resulting in a psychological disorder which can affect self-care behaviors (Tait & Chibnall, 2014). Psychosocial stressors include personal, cultural and religious beliefs, lack of understanding about the seriousness of the disease, the scarce and unavailable resources or the lack of self-care efficacy to manage the disease (Montague, Nichols, & Dutta, 2005).

There is overwhelming evidence in the literature suggesting that psychosocial barriers and interpersonal factors can impede self-care of diabetes or diabetes-related quality of life (Glasgow, Toobert, & Gillett, 2001). Psychosocial factors such as self-care efficacy are influenced by personal characteristics, social groups, societal and cultural influences (Glasgow, 1997). Glasgow, Toobert, & Gillette (2016) identified self-care efficacy, depression, health beliefs, and personal illness as examples of the psychological constructs; and stress and support from friends and close family members as interpersonal social factors that can impede diabetes self-care.

Self-care efficacy is a concept that was derived from the Social Cognitive Theory (SCT) in 1986 by Albert Bandura. The theory posits that "learning occurs in a social context with a dynamic and reciprocal interaction of the person, environment, and behavior". Many researchers of self-care efficacy have found the theory effective in promoting health behavior in people with various chronic illnesses. However, other researchers of diabetes have reported mixed results with the perceived effectiveness of self-care efficacy in the diabetes care, while Wengberg (2008) have suggested that self-care efficacy in the self-care process may function as a moderator to influence behavior change in people with diabetes (Lorig et al., 2010).

Chakkalakal et al. investigated the effectiveness in gender differences among 248 women (60.49 %) and 162 men (39.51 %) to determine the major CVD risk factors associated with low-income men and women with T2DM. The results showed diabetes self-care efficacy was significantly lower among females (Perceived Diabetes Self-management Scale score of 24.08 ± 5.63 *vs.* 25.50 ± 5.84, $p=0.01$) for male participants even though the female participants reported a longer duration of onset of Type II diabetes (9.62 ± 7.14 years *vs.* 7.87 ± 6.76 years, $p=0.01$) for male participants. There were no significant differences in demographic characteristics among the participants (Abstract from the 38th Annual Meeting of the Society of General Internal Medicine).

Diabetes is defined by the Expert Committee on the Diagnosis and Classification of Diabetes Mellitus as a "group of metabolic diseases characterized by hyperglycemia resulting from defects in insulin secretion, insulin action, or both" (p. 1). Diabetes is characterized by two broad etiopathogenetic categories - insulin-dependent diabetes mellitus (T1DM) and non-insulin dependent mellitus (T2DM). T1DM accounts for roughly 10% of the diabetes population and is more prevalent in non-Hispanic whites. T2DM accounts for over 90% of all cases of diabetes and is more prevalent in African-Americans, the elderly and other minorities. In T1DM, the body does not make the insulin needed to take up glucose from the blood; therefore, the patient must rely on synthetic insulin to control blood their sugar. In T2DM the body does not process the insulin it produces effectively; therefore, the patient must rely on oral medications to control their blood sugar.

Although some forms of diabetes has no known etiologies, researchers have associated the disease with genetic factors such as race, age, family history, stress, body mass index, and environmental factors such as drugs and toxins. Type I diabetes accounts for roughly 10% of the diabetes population and its etiology is characterized by the autoimmune destruction of the β cells causing insulin deficiency which ultimately results in hyperglycemia with ketoacidosis. Symptoms marked by hyperglycemia include blurred vision, excess urination, rapid weight loss, polyuria and polydipsia (Tull & Roseman, 2005).

Unlike T1DM which is a genetic malformation of the pancreatic islets or β cell destruction, T2DM is heavily influenced by insulin resistance and β cell dysfunction, environmental etiologic factors such as race/ethnicity, age, sedentary lifestyle, obesity, socioeconomic status (SES), and physical inactivity which results in insulin secretory defect. Diabetes is mostly acquired by one of three methods – genetic, behavioral, or environmental etiologic factors (Expert Committee on the Diagnosis and Classification of Diabetes Mellitus, 2003). Genetic factors are to a larger extent associated with the autoimmune pathologic processes occurring in the pancreatic islets. Behavioral factors are nonpharmacologic psychosocial issues that are influenced by lifestyle changes, social and cultural belief systems, or socioeconomic conditions.

Both T1DM and T2DM can be triggered by environmental factors such as food and nutrition, toxins, and pesticides such as Heptachlor which is commonly found in food and can easily pass in breast milk to infants (Patel, Bhattacharya, & Butte, 2010). Middle-aged Black/African-American women are generally predisposed to T2DM because of their genetic composition. T2DM occurs more frequently in women with previous gestational diabetes mellitus and individuals with dyslipidemia (high cholesterol), hypertension, and among certain racial/ethnic subgroups. T2DM is more prevalent in people aged 40 years and older. One of the known etiologies of T2DM is that its form can take many years to manifest and show classic symptoms because the hyperglycemia develops gradually putting the individuals at increased risk for microvascular and macrovascular complications (The Expert Committee on the Diagnosis and Classification of Diabetes Mellitus, 2003).

One of the most common risk factors for T2DM among middle-aged Black/African-American women is obesity. Obesity is measured as body mass index (BMI ≥30) (NIH, 2017). The high prevalence of obesity in the U.S has been termed a major public health epidemic because of its association with chronic illnesses such as T2DM, stroke, hypertension, some cancers, and heart disease (Barrington et al, 2007). In the U.S., the estimated cost of treating obesity-related diseases in 2010 was $190 billion (CDC, 2017). The association of obesity and T2DM in African-American women relative to their non-Hispanic white counterparts has long being established even after controlling for age, socioeconomic factors, and adiposity (Tull & Roseman, 2005). Research shows that more than 80% of people with diabetes are obese or overweight (Robert Wood Johnson Foundation) (RWJF, 2017).

The incidence of obesity-related cases in Texas is increasing and is more likely to predict increases in chronic illnesses such as diabetes and hypertension and result in adverse behavioral and psychosocial issues. According to the Texas Department of State Health Services Behavioral Risk Factor Surveillance System (BRFSS), the incidence of obesity rates increased from 10.7% in 1990 to 33.0% in 2017. Obesity is more profound among minorities and middle-aged adults. Based on the current trend, roughly 20 million or 75% of Texas adults could be obese or overweight by 2040.

In a survey conducted by (RWJF, 2016), Texas ranks 14th among the nation in adult obesity with roughly 33.0% of adults reported as obese. Middleaged adults (45 – 64 years of age) are reportedly more obese (39.2 %) compared to 30.6% of the elderly aged 65 years and older. African-Americans living in Texas are disproportionately obese (39.8 %) compared to other demographics, and more men (32.1 %) are obese than their female counterparts (33.9 %). Nationally, the obesity rates are similar to those in Texas. According to the National Center for Health Statistics (NCHS), the prevalence of obesity among African-American women is 56.9% compared with 37.5% for their AfricanAmerican male counterparts. There is a statistically significant difference in obesity rates between African-American women and non-Hispanic white women (35.5%) and Asian women (11.9%, NCHS, 2016).

Identifying African-American women with adverse psychosocial deficits towards self-care behaviors in the early stages of diagnosis may have practical implications in the way interventions are created to target the underlying causes and prevent further complications. The implication for this study may ascertain perceptions about barriers to self-care behaviors and may influence patient adherence and self-care efficacy for self-care behaviors, ultimately leading to better glycemic control.

Historical Overview

The concept and definitions of self-care over the past decades has evolved into a broad and multidimensional phenomenon shaped by many different domains of health including mental, social, physical, and psychological health. Over the decades, various terms have emerged for the phenomena such as selfcare, self-care management, and self-management all of which refer to the patient engaging in activities to optimize their own health. However, there is no general consensus on the definition of the concept.

The term "self-care" has been widely associated with an individual's ability to care for oneself in order to optimize their health (Richard & Shea, 2011). Barlow et al. (2002) describes self-care as the individual's ability to manage the symptoms, treatment, physical and psychological consequences associated with lifestyle changes inherent in living with a chronic condition. Selfcare, however, is not a new phenomenon in disease management.

The concept has been in practice from the beginning of time as people with acute or chronic illnesses have always engaged in activities in support of their own health and quality of life. Therefore, the origins of self-care can only be speculated. Epidemiological factors show that a "shift in disease patterns from acute to chronic disease makes self-care both a logistical necessity and an appropriate strategy" (Levin, 1983, p. 190). Conceptually, any activity a patient engages in outside the domain of a professional caregiver is considered self-care (Webber, Guo, & Mann, 2013).

Many different theoretical perspectives and paradigms have emerged that have been tested and translated into various health care models used in nursing and related healthcare practices. In 1959, Dorthea Orem, a nurse from Baltimore, Maryland proposed three inter-related theories of self-care: theory of self-care, theory of self-care deficit, and theory of nursing systems. According to Orem, self-care is a behavior initiated or performed by individuals on their own behalf to save life and promote health (Orem, 1990). The concept of self-care encapsulates personal attributes such as positive attitudes, knowledge, skills, determination, courage, and optimism to care for self and improve health (Akintola, 2001).

Orem's theory of self-care focuses on the self (1990), the "human's ability or power to engage in self-care and is affected by basic conditioning factors" (p. 49) which she referred to as self-care agency. Orem's theory, however, is based on the premise that people that are ill have the innate ability to care for themselves. However, when the self-care demand exceeds the individual's capacity to care for self, that person experiences a self- care deficit and thus have a need for nursing care (Orem, 1990).

The increasing prevalence of chronic illnesses, the advances in medical science and technology, and the proliferation of healthcare costs has contributed to a paradigm shift in disease management. Various healthcare policies began to emerge from governments and third-party payers to encourage individuals to be involved in their health care by accepting some of the responsibility for their own health.

In 1960s, the concept of self-management emerged in a book written on rehabilitation of chronically ill children by Thomas Creer and colleagues at *The Children's Research Asthma Institute and Hospital* in conjunction with their pediatric Asthma program. The term self-management which is similar in attributes to self-care is defined differently in a variety of health settings to indicate that the patient is an active participant in their own health care (Creer, Rene, & Christian, 1976).

Since 1983, the definition of "self-care" has evolved considerably to explain the process of enhancing one's involvement in their own health. Subsequent to the World Health Organization (WHO) definition in 1983, and on the occasion of World Health Day, a final definition of self-care emerged in 2013 to describe self-care as "the ability of individuals, families and communities to promote health, prevent disease, and maintain health and to cope with illness and disability with or without the support of a health-care provider" (Webber, Guo, & Mann, 2010, p. 1).

Empirical Research on Key Variables and/ or Constructs Self-care Management

Diabetes is a complex chronic condition that affects individuals uniquely. Diabetes self-care behavior is an important factor in the disease management process as it involves a multi-component of self-care activities like healthy dietary intake, glucose monitoring and insulin administration, all of which are lifestyle changing events (Cosansu & Erdogan, 2014). Self-care activities requires people to constantly monitor and maintain targeted blood glucose levels, adhere to medication regimen, maintain a certain weight, engage in regular exercises, and be compliant with medical checkups. In addition to maintaining targeted blood glucose levels, individuals with diabetes must monitor and control their blood pressure and lipid levels (Poolsup, Suksomboon, & Kyaw, 2013). Research shows that the consequences of diabetes can result into other serious comorbid conditions such as retinopathy, neuropathy, nephropathy, and heart disease (van der Heijden et al., 2012). This in turn can increase the likelihood for peripheral amputations, blindness, and kidney failure which can ultimately result in poorer health outcomes, diminished quality of life, and higher health care costs.

The Institute of Management (IOM) defines self-care management as "the systematic provision of education and supportive interventions by health care staff to increase patients' skills and confidence in managing their health problems, including regular assessment of progress and problems, goal setting, and problemsolving support" (IOM, 2003, p.144). Diabetes self-care management encompasses the concepts of self-care, patient empowerment, patient education, integrated disease management, motivational interviewing, and health coaching. Achieving these objectives requires appropriate diabetes self-care behaviors education (DSME) and adherence to self-care recommendations, which is the basis for acquiring and promoting knowledge particularly among people with diabetes.

Self-management support programs are widespread in chronic disease management. One of the most widely effective DSME programs is the Stanford Chronic Disease Self-management Program (CDSMP). Franek (2013) conducted a systematic review of 10 studies comprising of ($n = 6,074$) participants with various chronic illnesses including diabetes, to assess the effectiveness of the Stanford CDSMP in self-care behaviors for people with chronic illnesses. The reviewers investigated four specific areas of self-management: health status outcomes, health behavior outcomes, self-care efficacy, and healthcare utilization outcomes. Healthcare knowledge was not assessed in the review. The reviewers found a small but statistically significant short-term improvement across all the health outcomes including self-care efficacy and health-related quality of life. However, the reviewers found no evidence of improvement in healthcare utilization with the CDSMP.

Another study conducted by Forjuoh et al. (2014) evaluated the effectiveness of the CDSMP on HbA1c levels on two groups – a group enrolled in a CDSMP ($n = 101$) and a control group ($n = 95$). The demographics was enrolled in a randomized control trial in the U.S. and consisted of 196 participants with a mean age of 57.6 ±10.9 years of which 36.4% were a mix of African-Americans and non-white Hispanics. The primary outcome of interest in the study was a change in HbA1c levels from randomization to 12 months.

The mean HbA1c level for the participants was 9.3% ± 1.6%. There was no statistically significant difference in mean HbA1c between the control and CDSMP groups. Roughly 92.9% were overweight with a mean BMI of 34.3 ±7.4 kg/m^2. Participants randomized to the CDSMP group were enrolled into a 6-week class-room based self-care behaviors program with the goal of increasing self-care efficacy to reduce healthcare utilization and decrease disease-related symptoms and complications.

After 12 months from baseline to follow-up, HbA1c levels fell by 0.559% for the CDSMP group and 0.576% for the control group ($p < .0001$). The only significant difference between the two groups was a higher rate of change of people within the control group checking their feet ($p = 0.02$). The researchers found no significant differences between people in the control group and the CDSMP group. Although statistically significant increases were found in self-care efficacy in this study, the impact of CDSMP on self-care behaviors yields mixed results. These results are consistent with several other studies in the literature where self-care efficacy was found to be statistically significant with self-care management (Zulman et al., 2012).

Zulman et al. (2012) used a longitudinal study to examine the effects of psychosocial attributes on self-care management of glycemic control for ($n = 1834$) adults 51 years and older. The study explored the cross-sectional relationship between psychosocial attributes (diabetes-related emotional distress, prioritization of diabetes, care understanding, and risk awareness) and selfmanagement, and glycemic control using the covariates (age, race, sex, income and education). Researchers used multivariate regression analysis and found a significant association between all the psychosocial attributes and self-care management, and diabetes-related emotional distress. Among the psychosocial attributes examined, self-care management had the strongest relationship with self-care efficacy (adj. coeff = 8.1, $p < 0.01$) and emotional distress (adj. coeff = - 4.1, $p < 0.01$).

Coyle, Francis, and Chapman (2013) conducted a systematic review of 32 studies to evaluate the effectiveness of diabetes self-management behaviors (medication adherence, self-monitoring blood glucose, diet, physical activity, and foot care) and whether the behaviors were sustainable over time. Researchers found that although people with diabetes undertook regular self-management activities; however, the level of activity varied widely. Medication adherence was reported as the highest of all self-care behaviors (70% to 99%). The other selfmanagement behaviors varied widely in response to environmental factors, such as access to and availability of medications which can influence medication adherence. The review of literature found African-American women with diabetes had a high compliance rate of 80% on adherence to medications, diet, and physical activity (Coyle, Francis, and Chapman, 2013), even though other studies have found lower compliance or lower adherence rates among African-Americans with diabetes (Chlebowy, Hood, & LaJoie, 2013).

The outcome of T2DM may be attributable to the ability of the patient to effectively manage the disease. Management of T2DM may be challenging based on the resources available to the patient. Barriers to effective self-care behaviors is affected by the lack of psychosocial support, knowledge of the disease, medication non-adherence, cultural beliefs, socioeconomic disparities, health disparities, and environmental factors (Chlebowy, Hood, & LaJoie 2013). The observed difficulties in complying with treatment regimen may have some ethnical undertone. Chlebowy, Hood, and LaJoie (2013) posit that African- Americans were more likely to be less compliant with self-care behaviors. Mathew, Gucciardi, De Melo, and Barata (2012) posited that there are significant gender differences in T2DM self-care behaviors experiences, in that males display a more positive outlook than females that may report fear and more depressive symptoms. In a study conducted by Wilkinson, Whitehead, and Ritchie (2014), the researchers argued that identification of barriers to self-care behaviors is an important prerequisite in finding and reducing the devastating effects of T2DM and the long-term complications associated with the disease.

According to Laranjo et al. (2015), interventions directed to the promotion of self-care behaviors could be one of the most effective ways of combating T2DM. Irrespective of the strategies and promotional efforts by healthcare professionals to encourage compliance in self-care and life-style changes, the specificity and outcome may depend on the ability and characteristics of the targeted population (Laranjo et al., 2015). The failure of patients to achieve glycemic control, as a treatment regimen may be an indication that self-care behavior principles formulated by healthcare providers may be inadequate.

The literature has explored other social and external factors that influence self-care behaviors process for people with T2DM. Hu et al. (2013), stated that patients may lack the intervention strategies to meet their needs because of their inability to understand or comprehend the disease. Low health literacy for instance has been correlated with poor glycemic control leading to complications among people of minority groups (Hu et al., 2013). This may be related to the level of participation of the patients during the treatment phase of the self-care behavior process.

One of the psychosocial factors that is known to impede the self-care process is depression. Depression is more prevalent in African-Americans and in women with and without diabetes than their non-Hispanic white counterparts (Fuentes & Aranda, 2012; Weinger, 2007). The onset of chronic illnesses has been identified as a major underlying cause for psychosocial dysfunctions. However, most interventions for diabetes have relied mainly on pharmacologic interventions. Certain non-pharmacologic interventions such as cognitive behavior therapy and motivational interviewing have been found to be effective in helping people cope with diabetes and diabetes-related complications (Weinger, 2007).

Most studies on behavioral issues related to glycemic control have focused primarily on depression (Weinger, 2007). In a meta-analysis review of the literature, Lustman and Gavard (2008) found that there were more psychosomatic interactions in people with diabetes than depression. People with diabetes require a high degree of self-care and significant lifestyle adjustments which includes daily monitoring of blood glucose levels, adhering to medication regimen, engaging in physical exercise, maintaining a reasonable body weight, modifying meal portions, and getting regular checkups. Adapting to these behavioral changes can increase the risk of mood and anxiety disorders which may later manifest into depression and other forms of psychosocial dysfunctions (Edge & Ellis, 2010).

A study reported by the World Health Organization (WHO) stated that psychosocial issues including depression, psychological distress, and anxiety affect women to a greater extent than men across different settings (WHO, 2017). A similar study published in the *Journal of Abnormal Psychology* by the American Psychological Association (APA, 2017) found that women were more likely to be diagnosed with depression or anxiety than did men. The *APA* also supported the assertion that women were more likely than men to suffer from depression because "women ruminate more frequently than men, focusing repetitively on their negative emotions and problems rather than engaging in more active problem solving" (APA, 2017, p. 1.). However, one study found that women were more likely to have better psychosocial adjustment to their illness than men did (Evangelista, Kagawa-Singer, and Dracup, 2001).

Depression is not a unique phenomenon in people with chronic illnesses. The prevalence of depression was observed in patients with diabetes more than 300 years ago by Dr. Thomas Willis, a British physician that associated diabetes with "sadness or long sorrow" (Edge & Ellis, 2009). Anderson, Freedland, Clouse, and Lustman (2001) conducted a systematic review of 21,351 people and found the prevalence of clinically relevant depression among people with diabetes was 31% and the prevalence of major depression in people with diabetes was 11%. One study found that "Coexisting depression in people with diabetes is associated with decreased adherence to treatment, poor metabolic control, higher complication rates, decreased quality of life, increased healthcare use and cost, increased disability and lost productivity, and increased risk of death" (Edge & Willis, 2009, p. 1.).

There is a plethora of literature that has associated depression and socioeconomic factors as examples of psychosocial dysfunctions that impede the effective management of diabetes among African-American women (Tull & Roseman, 2005). There is also a scarcity of literature that has examined the psychosocial stressors that significantly contributes to impede the effective management of the disease among middle-aged Black/African-American women with diabetes (Tull & Roseman, 2005). Egede, Grubaugh, and Ellis (2010) posited that 42.5% of women with diabetes were suffering from major depression while 38.4% within the same group had minor depression severe enough to require treatment. Glasgow (1997) posit that some behavior specific patterns that people with diabetes want to change are self-care efficacy, health beliefs, problemsolving skills (knowledge), and distress. Anderson et al. (2001) found a substantial increase in the prevalence of diabetes-related distress among people with diabetes compared to the general adult population.

A body of literature has associated depressive symptoms with diabetes. Poulsen and Pachana (2012) found that patients with T2DM disproportionately experience anxiety, depressive symptoms, depression and symptoms of psychological disorder leading to poor quality of life than the general population. A review of the literature revealed several factors such as lifestyles, socioeconomic factors, obesity and stressful life to be associated with diabetes (Windle & Windle, 2013). Relatively, people with a history of lifetime depression has been shown to be closely associated with worsen blood glucose leading to diabetes or diabetes-related complications (de Groot, Kushnick, Doyle, Merrill, McGlynn, Shubrook, & Schwartz, 2010). Charteris-Black (2012) posited the rate of depression in women is twice that of men and Windle and Windle (2013) stated that individuals with T2DM were more likely to experience depression than those without the disease. Individuals with T2DM have more depression and depressive symptoms leading to higher complications and functional disabilities compared to patients without diabetes (Dismuke & Egede, 2010). This rising statistics of depression among individuals with diabetes may be one of the reasons the American Diabetes Association continually modify the guidelines to recommend mandatory screening for adults with diabetes (Bogner, Morales, Vries, & Cappola, 2012).

The relationship between depression and poor self-care behaviors for people with diabetes is well documented in the literature (Weinger, 2007). In one study, Lustman and Gavard (2000) conducted a meta-analysis review of 30 studies in the literature and found depression was significantly associated with poor glycemic control and hyperglycemia. The researchers suggested that based on clinical data, there appears to be a reciprocal association between depression and hyperglycemia; meaning that hyperglycemia may also be a consequence of depression or vice versa (Weinger, 2007). Lerman et al. (2004) and Park et al. (2004) also confirmed the assertion that depression affects a patient's ability to self-manage their chronic illnesses.

According to Stoop, Spek, Pop, and Pouwer (2011), depression and anxiety are among the psychosocial stressors associated with ineffective self-care and poor glycemic control in people with T2DM. The increased risk for these conditions could lead to micro vascular and macro vascular (hypertension, hyperlipidemia, obesity, and sedentary lifestyle) outcomes further leading to heart disease or morbidity.

There is empirical evidence suggesting that middle-aged Black/African-American women with diabetes have a greater risk for the chronic complications associated with diabetes than their non-Hispanic white counterparts (Egede & Gogo-Jack, 2005; Mayer-Davis et al., 2009), particularly for diabetic nephropathy (Crook & Patel, 2004; Mayer-Davis et al., 2009).

A body of research has explored the effects of psychosocial attitudes in diabetes self-care behaviors. Kato et al. (2016) conducted a study of 26 adult patients aged 30 to 64 years old with T2DM to examine how patients "psychologically and behaviorally respond to internalized stigma through social stigma." Researchers found that participants with T2DM tend to internalize stigma, which can lead to social distance attitudes and hinder the degree of compliance with their treatment regimen, and also question their sense of selfworth. Stigma refers to "attitudes and beliefs that lead people to reject, avoid, or fear those they perceive as being different". Stigma internalizing is associated with depression, social anxiety, and somatization. Stigma can adversely harm individuals in several ways – it can exacerbate chronic illnesses such as diabetes, it can precipitate social isolation which can lead to manifestations of distress and psychosocial disorder, and it can hinder adherence to treatment regimen (Anna et al., 2016).

Zulman et al. (2012) argued that feeling of emotion distress during the treatment process of T2DM, worrying about blood sugar level or paying for the medications needed to treat the disease may lead to discouragement during the treatment process which may influence the health outcome. The psychosocial burden of diabetes self-care is not fully understood, but deeper understanding of psychosocial behavior in relation to diabetes self-care is necessary to address the barrier to self-care behaviors for people with T2DM (Nicolucci et al., 2013). Though psychosocial factors play a role in T2DM self-care behaviors (Cosansu & Erdogan, 2014), gaps exist in the explanation of association between psychosocial attitudes and the knowledge and support required to achieve outcome expectations (Nicolucci et al., 2013). Relatively, research shows that one of the most important psychosocial factors is perceived self-care efficacy, which is a construct of the HBM that explains the belief of an individual's capability to manage individual situation to achieve an expected outcome (Rosenstock, 1974).

Self-care Knowledge

Self-care knowledge is a pre-requisite to appropriately self-manage diabetes disease for a positive outcome. Ahola and Groop (2012) argued that lack of knowledge is a top tier of the list of investigative studies to evaluate barrier to self-care behaviors during the disease treatment process. According to Al-Qazaz et al. (2011), higher diabetes knowledge is a significant predictor of good glycemic control which is one of the precursors for effective self-care behaviors of T2DM. Patient's knowledge of diabetes could help in the administration of insulin during the self-care process or self-reporting of health status process of the treatment regimen. During the diagnostic and treatment phase of T2DM, healthcare professionals often require patients to report their health status to the medical providers to enable adequate treatment planning. The patient's ability to comply with the instructions may be highly dependent on the disease knowledge. Fan et al. (2016) posited that health literacy is needed for quality improvement in patient care, as limited disease knowledge may be associated with poor glycemic control and complications in diabetes patients.

Another implication of poor diabetes knowledge may be related to a patient's ability to understand or use health information that may be beneficial to them and could determine treatment outcome. Diabetes knowledge could be derived from health promotion pamphlets and health awareness programs. This process of information dissemination could be challenging if the targeted population lack the educational capacity to understand the recommendations and preventative measures. Hook-Anderson et al. (2015) in a Diabetes Prevention Program study found that lifestyle education on T2DM prevention or delay was an effective intervention across racial and ethnic groups. Educational programs designed to intervene and educate patients in the treatment of T2DM may be complex depending on the theoretical models and the related skills of the instructor (Steinsbekk et al., 2012), but good quality education and psychosocial interventions may be of benefit to the patients during the treatment process.

Dussa, Parimalakrishnan, and Sahay (2015) conducted a study to assess self-care knowledge in (N = 80) patients between 18 years and 85 years with T2DM at Osmania Hospital, Hyderabad, India. The aim of the study was to assess self-care knowledge using the diabetes knowledge questionnaire (DKQ) and to determine its correlation with HbA1c levels. To answer the research question, the researchers used a quantitative, non-experimental cross-sectional study with a correlational design. Quantitative analysis was used in the study to collect specific questions about the participants and to collect numeric data using survey questionnaires. Quantitative analysis was used to determine the mean age of the participants and the mean of the HbA1c levels. Using statistical analysis, the researchers found a significant correlation between HbA1c levels and disease duration.

A similar study by Groh and Moran (2017) conducted a descriptive, bivariate, correlation analyses with a cross-sectional design study using n=30 primarily minority patients with a mean age of 57.9 years and have T2DM. The dependent variable was glycemic control and the independent variables were selfcare efficacy and depression. The study found no significant relationship between depression and HbA1c but found a significant inverse relationship between depression and self-care efficacy. The non-significant findings between glycemic control and depression is inconsistent with many studies in the literature that have suggested a significant relationship between these two variables.

Cani, Lopes, Queiroz, and Nery (2015) conducted a randomized controlled trial of 70 adults with T2DM aged 45 years and older. The objective of the study was to evaluate the impact of a clinical pharmacy program on health outcomes on patients with T2DM receiving insulin therapy at a teaching hospital in Brazil. Patients were enrolled into the program if they were diagnosed with T2DM and had an HbA1c $\geq$ 8.0%. Two groups were created: the intervention group (IG, n = 34) and the control group (CG, n = 36).

The primary outcome measure was change in HbA1c measures and the secondary outcome measures were change in self-reported medication adherence, medication knowledge, home blood glucose monitoring techniques, insulin injection techniques, and self-reported diabetes health-related qualify of life. The IG received a diabetes education protocol on acute and chronic complications and the significance of lifestyle changes involving diet, physical activity, and smoking cessation). The CG only received the regular treatment without the benefits of the education protocol provided to the IG.

The outcome measures (medication adherence, medication knowledge, home blood glucose monitoring techniques, insulin injection techniques, and selfreported diabetes health-related qualify of life) were evaluated at baseline and at 6 months follow-up. All the outcome measures significantly improved in the IG but remained unchanged in the CG. The primary outcome measure HbA1c significantly improved in the IG from a baseline m 9.78±1.55 SD to a 6-month follow-up final with a m 9.21±1.41 SD ($p < 0.001$) but remained unchanged in the CG - m 9.61±1.38 SD vs. 9.53±1.68 SD ($p > 0.999$). The change in HbA1c measures decreased significantly by 0.57%, which is consistent with other studies in the literature. Diabetes knowledge also improved significantly in the IG from a m 9.91±2.69 SD to a m 15.74±3.03 SD ($p < 0.001$). Medication knowledge increased in the IG from a m 4.47±0.84 SD to a m 6.58±1.29 SD ($p < 0.001$).

Self-care Efficacy

Self-care efficacy represents "an individual's confidence for implementing behavior change based on efficacy beliefs and outcome expectation" (Ryan et al., 2013, p. 266). Bowen et al. (2015) postulated that higher levels of self-care efficacy in disease management may be associated with self-motivation, self-empowerment and self-confidence in a patient's ability to influence disease outcome during the treatment. Self-care efficacy is a critical predictor of numerous health behaviors. Several studies have postulated that selfcare efficacy could be associated with better quality of life for most adults with chronic illnesses. According to Ryan et al. (2013), diet, physical exercise, and behavior change may be sufficient to suggest that self-care efficacy in self-care behaviors is important for treatment outcome in people with T2DM.

Cummings et al. (2017) conducted a post-hoc analysis of prospective, randomized, controlled trial of 129 middle-aged Black/African-American women with uncontrolled diabetes in rural southeastern U.S. The objective was to determine whether diabetes-related emotional distress was associated with lower poor glycemic control, inadequate self-care behaviors, and medication adherence among rural African-American women with uncontrolled T2DM. After a 12month follow-up from baseline, researchers found a significant improvement in HbA1c levels, self-care activities, self-care efficacy, and medication adherence. Changes in diabetes-related distress were also significantly and inversely associated with increases in self-care efficacy and improvements in medication adherence and self-care behaviors.

Researchers have shown that treating T2DM involves a lifelong process of learning and effective self-care behaviors including insulin administration, medication adherence, dietary changes and exercise. For example, Oftedal, Bru, and Karlsen (2011) found that activities such as exercise are a necessary component to achieve adequate metabolic control in order to avoid long-term complications. As one of the factors for preventing or managing T2DM is exercise, Bosch, Robbins, and Anderson (2015) recommended at least 150 minutes per week of moderate -intensity physical activities to achieve health related benefit of diabetes treatment. T2DM can also be treated by increased physical activities to reduce disease complications. The beliefs and capability of the individual to enhance metabolic control could reduce certain risks that may lead to complications of T2DM (van der Heijden et al., 2012). Olson and McAuley (2015) posited that a critical disease intervention factor such as physical activity could be a first-line therapy to control the progression of T2DM.

Mehta et al. (2015) conducted a cross-sectional study of 126 women with T2DM in India to determine whether low levels of self-efficacy were responsible for the lack of diabetes knowledge and increase in prevalence of T2DM among rural Indian women. used the Michigan Diabetes Empowerment scale, Knowledge scale, and Attitudes and Assessment Practices scale. The mean knowledge score was 10.77±2.866 out of 24 points. Using age-adjusted multiple regression analysis, researchers found a statistically significant positive correlation between diabetes knowledge and self-efficacy ($p < .001$).

Individual efficacy is a major component of disease self-care practices. There is a plethora of literature on exercise efficacy for people with T2DM. For example, Park and Lee (2015) investigated the effects of exercise on glycemic control using data from 1,328 patients aged 30 to 90 years, on the Korean Health and Nutrition Examination Survey database. Using linear and logistic regression methods to analyze the data, researchers found that engaging in low to moderate intensity aerobic exercise such as walking for 150 minutes spread over a three day period could potentially be beneficial and lower the risk of glycemic control failure by 0.248 times (95% CI: 0.084–0.734, $p < 0.05$). Researchers also found waist circumference, duration of diabetes, presence of hypertension; medication adherence, physical activity, and income level were significantly associated with lowering glycemic control ($p<.05$). Another study by Selvin et al. (2004) cited in Park and Lee (2015) posited that a 1% reduction in HbA1c could decrease the risk of cardiovascular complications by 15 to 20% in individuals with T2DM. The ADA recommends moderate to rigorous aerobic exercise each week spread over a three-day period.

A major risk factor for diabetes is diet and nutrition. However, dietary practices are mainly influenced by cultural backgrounds. Diet and nutrition plays a significant role in managing obesity and diabetes. There is a body of knowledge in the literature indicating that obesity is a major risk factor for T2DM and diabetes-related complications (Sharma & Lau, 2013). Obesity is characterized as a physical and psychological problem. The etiological factors of obesity are associated with psychosocial, environmental, and genetic attributes. For example, people who live in a "toxic environment" in which access to physical activity is limited or calorically dense foods are readily available are more likely to have difficulty controlling their consumption of food, exercising, or maintaining a healthy weight (Collins & Bentz, 2009, p. 1).

Koote et al. (2012) characterized obesity as a metabolic disorder believed to have developed by a combination of lifestyle changes and genetic susceptibility. Moreno-Indias et al. (2014) asserted that obesity and T2DM are metabolic risk profiles associated with the presence of low-grade inflammatory component in the tissue involving the regulation of metabolism in the body systems. Ning et al. (2013) reported that a positive family history of diabetes and obesity are precursors and risk factors for developing T2DM.

One study by Khan et al. (2016) examined the association between obesity, diabetes, and aggressiveness of prostate cancer in a cross-sectional study of 991 African-Americans and 1,058 White Americans. Researchers found overall, diabetes was not associated with prostate cancer aggressiveness (OR 1.04; 95% CI 0.79 - 1.37). However, researchers found obesity, independent of diabetes was positively associated with high aggressive prostate cancer in White Americans (OR 1.98; 95% CI 1.14 - 3.43), but not in African-Americans (OR 1.09; 95% CI 0.71 - 1.67).

Garg, Maurer, Reed, and Selagamsetty (2014) conducted a multi metaanalysis of case control studies and prospective cohort studies of the relationship between obesity, diabetes, and cancer. Researchers found a body of evidence supporting the assertion that there is an association between diabetes (particularly T2DM), cancer, and obesity. There found evidence in the literature that T2DM is an independent risk factor for several types of cancers including liver, pancreas, breast, bladder, colorectal, endometrial, and Hodgkin lymphoma, with hepatocellular carcinoma cancer being the biggest risk of all (see Figure 2.).

However, researchers did not find any evidence of a positive association between diabetes and prostate cancer. The researchers did find a statistically positive association between obesity and pancreatic cancer. The negative association increased with increases in the duration of diabetes and is based on the finding that "insulin is positively associated with the growth of both normal and cancerous prostate cells" (p. 98). As a result, decreased insulin production that is typically seen in people with diabetes, may inhibit the growth of prostate cancer cells. As shown in Figure 3, Hepatocellular carcinoma (RR 2.54; 95% CI 1.9 – 3.2), Endometrium (RR 2.2; 95% CI 1.8 – 2.7) and Pancreatic (RR 1.9; 95% CI 1.5 – 2.5) are the biggest risks for people with diabetes.

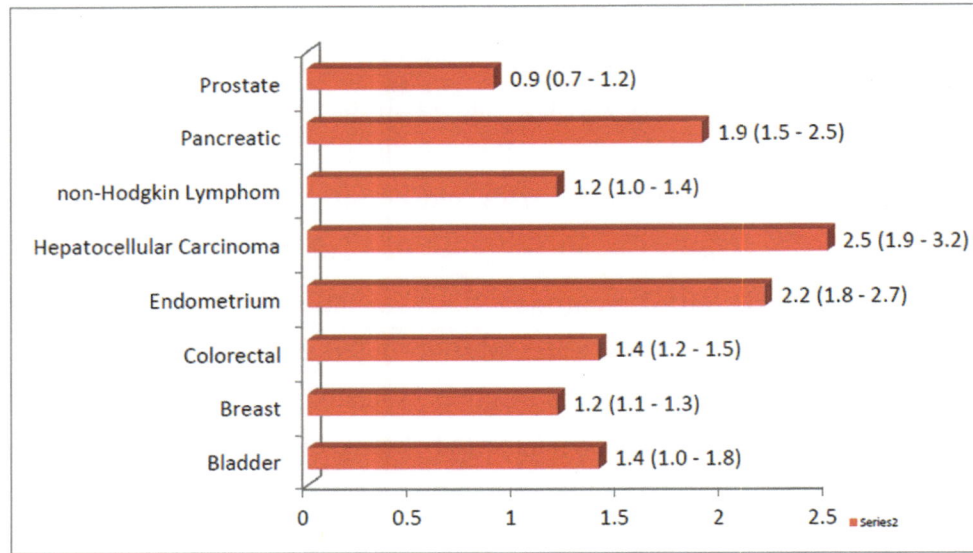

Figure 3. Diabetes as a Risk Factor for Certain Cancer Types (RR[95%CI]). (Yeh et al., 2015).

Sami, Ansari, Butt, and Hamid (2017) conducted a review of several studies of T2DM and self-management behaviors among various ethnicities in Saudi Arabia and Qatar. The researchers reviewed specific areas of self-care behavior (physical activity, attitude towards diet, and knowledge of self-care) and found a commonality of self-care deficits among ethnically diverse patients with T2DM. Most self-care deficits were found in patients attitudes towards noncompliance with dietary and physical exercise behaviors, which are major risk factors for T2DM.

In one example, researchers found Saudis consumed too many high sugary drinks, ate more red meat and fried foods, are overweight, and live a sedentary lifestyle. A comparable attitude and behavior was found in people with diabetes in Qatar that shares similar traditions and customs with the Saudi culture. Two other studies assessed knowledge of the effects of diet on diabetes among both Qatari and Saudi patients. The Qatari study found half of the patients were significantly deficient in diabetes knowledge while the Saudi study found 97.3% of males and 93.1% of females had less knowledge of the significance of monitoring their diabetes. In the Japanese culture, researchers found an increased risk of association between T2DM and elevated intake of white rice among Japanese women (Sami, Ansari, Butt, & Hamid, 2017).

Teixeira et al. (2015) conducted a systematic review of 35 studies testing 42 putative mediators for identifying successful outcomes in obesity and weight control treatment. The study reviewed specific mediators (self-regulatory and psychological mechanisms) and their association with self-care behaviors (diet, physical activity, and weight change). The review looked at the short (<12 months) and long-term (> 12 months) effects of mediators on self-care behaviors. The outcome of the review indicated limited evidence of self-care efficacy, selfregulation, and autonomous motivation as mediators of favorable weight control and physical activity outcomes. However, the review found long-term, self-care efficacy was unrelated as a mediator of dietary intake. These results were consistent across 75% of the studies reviewed. The review did not assess whether self-care efficacy and self-regulation were independent of self-care knowledge.

Bosomworth (2013) reported that obesity and T2DM together are a combination of risk factors that can increase cardiometabolic disorder in individuals leading to the development of cardiovascular diseases. In a study conducted by XU et al. (2017), the researchers found that the risk of diabetes is attributed to obesity, which is closely associated with poor liver function that may influence deficient insulin production and ultimately complicate the diabetes process. Taken together, obesity can cause insulin resistance or deficient insulin production in the body, which may lead to the development of T2DM. The rising number of obesity among adults is causing a major concern in the healthcare sector as this metabolic disorder have risk factors that are closely associated with T2DM (Moreno-Indias et al., 2014).

The socioeconomic impact of diabetes on the U.S. economy is staggering. Studies show that 1 in 5 healthcare dollars in the U.S. is spent on treating diabetes. The estimated cost of treating diabetes and its complications in the U.S. in 2012 was $245 billion of which $176 billion is attributed to direct medical costs and $69 billion is attributed to lost productivity. The medical cost of treating people with diabetes is 2.3 times higher than those without the disease. The average medical expenditures incurred for people with diabetes is $13,700 of which $7,900 is directly attributable to the disease. The largest component of the medical expenditures (43%) is attributed to hospital inpatient care.

The cost of treating diabetes imposes a substantial burden on societal and community resources. Nationwide, the lost productivity from the inability to work due to disease-related disability is roughly $21.6 billion. Roughly $18.5 billion is attributed to lost productive capacity due to early mortality (ADA, 2013). Worldwide, the estimated cost of treating diabetes and its complications exceeded $376 billion in 2010 and is projected to exceed $490 billion by 2030 (International Diabetes Federation [IDF], 2012).

In Texas, the cost burden of treating T2DM is substantially higher than the other ranking states. The cost of treating both T1DM and T2DM was over $1.77 billion in 2010 of which T2DM accounted for $1.45 billion (82%) and 223,855 hospital stays. Middle-aged adults accounted for 105,870 (47%) hospital stays. Females accounted for $727,708,828 (42%) and African-Americans accounted for $349,216,500 (20%). Dallas and Harris counties contributed substantially to the rising cost of diabetes treatment, accounting for $846,782,272 (49%) (BRFSS, 2010).

Several studies have associated the onset of T2DM in African-Americans, with socioeconomic factors (education, income, occupation). Earlier studies on the subject of diabetes suggested that the frequency of diabetes among African Americans and White Americans decrease with increasing levels of education and family income (Tull & Roseman, 2005). This suggests that a rise in educational levels and family incomes may increase the timely and affordable access to healthcare, and potentially decrease the risks and incidence of chronic illnesses.

Osborn, Mayberry, Wagner, and Welch (2014) posited that racial or ethnic minorities may be vulnerable to diabetes as a result of their low socioeconomic status and the inability to afford transportation to or pay for medical care. Researchers referred to this phenomenon as a cumulative stressor where individuals with low income or low economic status experience overlapping vulnerability to disease agent and a low quality of life. For instance, people from low socioeconomic status are more likely to experience non-adherence to their medications or lack access to quality healthcare and treatments. As a result, this many trigger psychological stressors that may result in depressive symptoms, low efficacy, and low self-esteem.

The Institute of Medicine (IOM) defines access to care as "the timely use of personal health services to achieve the best health outcomes" (IOM, 1993, p. 1.). Prior to the enactment of the Affordable Care Act ("ACA") of 2010, in 2009 roughly 85% of middle-aged adults (45 – 64 years old) were less likely to have health insurance. The Medical Expenditure Panel Survey found in 2008, middleaged adults were more likely to have out-of-pocket medical expenses and health insurance premiums that were more than 10% of total family income. Health insurance facilitates access to medical care. Studies have shown that uninsured individuals were more likely to delay getting access to care, have their diagnosis at later disease stages, receive less quality care and become sicker when hospitalized, spend more days hospitalized and are likely to die during hospitalization (Agency for Healthcare Research and Quality (AHRQ), 2017).

In 2010, the U.S. Congress enacted the Affordable Care Act (ACA) which comprises two pieces of legislation – the Patient Protection and Affordable Care Act (2010) and the Health Care and Education Reconciliation Act (2010). The objective of the ACA was to expand coverage to all Americans, hold insurance companies accountable, lower healthcare costs, guarantee more choices, and enhance the quality of care for all Americans.

The ACA provided a provision to expand Medicaid coverage to millions of low-income families including people that had limited access to employerbased coverage and individuals that had limited income below 133 percent of the Federal Poverty Level (FPL) to purchase coverage on their own. The provision was through a combination of Medicaid expansion, premium tax credits, or private insurance reforms (CMS, 2016). The ACA had the potential to reach over 47 million Americans that lack health insurance coverage as well as millions more that were underinsured or lack the finances to purchase their own healthcare insurance.

The direct benefit of the ACA to middle-aged Black/African-American women with low to moderate income was a reduction in healthcare disparities, elimination of the requirements for preexisting conditions, capping annual out-ofpocket spending, widening the pool of health insurance exchanges, increasing coverage for preventive screenings, and improving better coordinated care. A portion of the benefits were intended to enable low and moderate income Americans, the uninsured, and underinsured to have access to quality health care under the Medicaid expansion program (CMS, 2016).

While the intent of the ACA was to provide coverage to all Americans, the June 2012 Supreme Court ruling made it optional for states to opt out of the program. As of 2015, 31 states including the

District of Columbia have adopted the Medicaid expansion program thereby providing health coverage or eligibility to millions of uninsured and high risk individuals. The state of Texas did not adopt the Medicaid expansion under the ACA (Kaiser Family Foundation ([KFF], 2016). However, many high risk individuals such as middle-aged Black/African American women have low SES status and are either without adequate health insurance or live in medically underserved areas. The effect of inadequate health coverage or the limited access to quality care may contribute to long term psychosocial and behavioral dysfunctions on self-care behaviors among the atrisk individuals.

Effective patient-provider communications is critical to the treatment process for people with T2DM. Researchers refer to T2DM as a life-changing episode for patients and the ability to communicate the prescribed medication regimen is a vital tool in the disease management process. During the counseling phase of the treatment process, healthcare providers may be considered part of the support group equipped with the communication skills to discuss the medication regimen to include past and future health behaviors (Mulder et al., 2015). From a bio psychosocial perspective, a well-tailored patient-centered communication approach may be needed to recommend self-care behaviors procedures to the diabetes patients (Mulder et al., 2015) to maximize medication adherence.

Individualized communication between the patient and healthcare provider may be important when discussing self-care behaviors such as monitoring of blood glucose for the successful coping with the challenges posed by diabetes treatment (Weymann et al., 2013). This process of targeted communication may help patient avoid barrier to treatment regimen. Diabetes education from a health provider's perspective could help patients avoid the common barriers to psychosocial behaviors such as self-care efficacy and social support as demonstrated by the Health Belief Model (HBM) used in this study. When viewed from a biopsychosocial approach, the common communication barriers between patients and healthcare providers such as nurses are lack of skills and self-care efficacy (Mulder et al., 2015).

Behavior modification may be a necessary factor in T2DM treatment following a diagnosis to avoid the risk of disease progression and complications (Mulder et al., 2015). Failure to engage the patient early in the onset of the disease to modify their behavior such as dietary intake, involvement in physical activities and blood glucose monitoring that may impact their quality of life could complicate the intervention process and may lead to the development of psychosocial barriers. For example, Weymann et al (2015) argued that patient's empowerment by providers through effective communication can be observed as a motivational construct, which may positively influence self-care behaviors as inherent capability of disease control to improve health outcomes. Researchers have noted that the ability of the patient to relate to the healthcare provider and make informed decisions based on the information shared could eliminate some barriers to self-care behaviors in T2DM treatment.

Diabetes Self-management Education

Diabetes Self-management Education is the process of facilitating knowledge, skills, and the ability for appropriate self-management behavior in people with diabetes. The knowledge acquired in-turn helps patients improve clinical outcomes and self-management behavior to reduce the risk of secondary complications associated with the disease (Funnell et al. (2010). For people with diabetes, a low HbA1c (<7%) is a good indicator of self-care management. Elevated levels of HbA1c are considered significant risk factors for complications in people with the disease, including cardiovascular risk factors, stroke, and microvascular and macrovascular complications (ADA, 2018).

Health disparities in endocrine diseases such as diabetes and its complications and morbidities have a higher prevalence among non-Hispanic Black populations than it does in white populations. Several researchers have examined the factors that influence poor self-care for individuals with diabetes. Spanakis and Golden (2013) noted in the literature that the factors contributing to poor self-care management of diabetes among minorities were biological, behavioral (depression, physical inactivity, poor control of blood pressure, inadequate self-monitoring of blood glucose), and social and environmental contributors such as the lack of access to health care and health care education.

Rickheim, Flader, Weaver, and Kendall (2002) conducted a study on 170 subjects with T2DM, to compare the effectiveness of delivering diabetes selfmanagement education in a group and individual setting. The participants received diabetes education over a 6 month period. The objective was to determine patients' attitudes, knowledge of diabetes, changes in self-care management behaviors, and medication adherence. Changes were assessed at baseline and after 2-weeks, 3-months, and 6-months during the education session. Both the individual and group settings reported improvements in knowledge, attitudes, and health-related quality of life, including other biological factors. Overall, the results showed that HbA1c decreased from 8.5±1.8% at baseline to 6.5±0.8% at 6 months ($p < 0.01$) among the population. There was a reduction of 1.7±1.9% among individual setting, and 2.5±1.8% among the group setting.

Gaps in the Literature

Diabetes is a chronic metabolic illness characterized by comorbidities, such as hypertension, obesity, and dyslipidemia. Cheng et al. (2012) postulated that adults with T2DM tend to have less knowledge of the disease. In spite of the similarities in pharmacologic interventions in the treatment of T2DM, AfricanAmericans are underrepresented in access to evidence-based non-pharmacologic self-care behaviors programs such as the CDSMP. This may be due in part to socio-cultural factors (racism, discrimination, lack of trust in the healthcare system, and unequal access to care) (Becker, Gates, & Newsom, 2004; Rooks & Whitfield, 2004; Dell & Whitman, 2011; Mingo, Eagle, & Lau, 2017). CDSMP programs help to enhance self-care efficacy and behavioral activation through patient education of people with chronic illnesses. The lack of knowledge and lifestyle modifications for some middle-aged Black/African-American women with T2DM can complicate disease progression and show manifestations of induced stress and depression. The effects of stress and depression and the emotional coping of dealing with a chronic illness through decreased self-care efficacy can have a deleterious impact on health outcomes.

The existing evidence that continues to be gathered on the benefits of increased self-care efficacy in managing chronic illnesses is mixed, at best and the relationship between confidence (self-care efficacy) and knowledge is sparse and demands considerable attention (Ludman et al., 2013). Although there is empirical evidence suggesting that psychosocial factors play a major role in achieving adequate results in self-care behaviors (Cosansu & Erdogan, 2014); however, gaps exist in the explanation of association between psychosocial attitudes and the knowledge required to achieve outcome expectations (Nicolucci et al., 2013). Boulware et al. (2009) conducted a cross-sectional study of 195 patients enrolled in randomized controlled trial on hypertension management. The objective was to identify predictors of perceptions, and correlate perceptions with adherence to high blood pressure management. Reseachers found race, gender, presence of diabetes mellitus, and knowledge were independent predictors of low perceived susceptibility to chronic kidney disease (CKD). This underscores the significance of the lack of knowledge of the potential health threat of CKD in people with diabetes and hypertension. It is this existing gap in knowledge and its relationship linking to self-care efficacy, self-care management of diabetes, and CDSMP that is the basis for this study.

Conclusion

This chapter reviewed the literature on the effectiveness of self-care efficacy, self-care knowledge, and self-care management as a tool in influencing psychosocial behaviors in middle-aged Black/African-American women living in north Texas with T2DM. The review of the literature showed that although there is a plethora of literature on behavioral issues associated with patient's ability to self-manage their T2DM, there is paucity of empirical research in psychosocial and behavioral attitudes in middle-aged Black/African-American women with T2DM. Research with some populations has indicated that self-care efficacy is not an effective tool in the self-care management process; however, many other studies that have investigated the phenomenon show a contrasting view point.

Summary

Chapter 2 included a review of literature discussing the relationship between self-care efficacy, self-care knowledge, and self-care management and how it influences the self-care process in middle-aged Black/African-American women with T2DM. In this chapter, the researcher explored the psychosocial factors that influence self-care efficacy, self-care knowledge, and self-care management using HBM. The chapter explored the concept of self-care efficacy as an important construct for T2DM and the patient's ability to achieve positive glycemic control. The psychosocial and physiological aspects as internal and external factors that contribute to self-care barriers to disease management and the related health outcome were mentioned. Literature discussing consequences of obesity and its associated disorders as precursor to the onset of T2DM were reviewed and the findings were presented. Although discussions of this behavioral inactivity and lifestyle changes were not exhaustive in this chapter, the independent risk factor and its metabolic dysfunctions were recognized as a genetic susceptibility to the development of diabetes. The methodology for the study including the scales of measure are discussed in the preceding chapter 3.

CHAPTER 3

Methodology

The purpose of this descriptive, quantitative, correlational study was to assess the association and magnitude of the relationship, if any, between diabetesrelated knowledge, self-care efficacy, and self-care management in middle-aged Black/African-American women (45 – 64 years of age) with T2DM in north Texas. Chapter 2 discussed the review of the literature regarding the relationship between self-care efficacy, self-care knowledge, and self-care management in middle-aged Black/African-American women with T2DM in north Texas. The HBM was presented as a conceptual framework to guide this study in an attempt to explain healthcare behaviors using the three variables self-care efficacy, selfcare knowledge, and self-care management.

Chapter 2 explored the concept of self-care efficacy as an important construct for T2DM and the patient's ability to achieve positive glycemic control. Chapter 3 presents the research methodology, research approach, research design including population and samples, instrumentation and operationalization of constructs, data collection procedures, plan for data analysis, threats to validity, and ethical concerns.

Research Approach Appropriateness

This study was a quantitative, non-experimental research with a correlational design. A quantitative or a qualitative design is feasible for this study. However, the quantitative method with a correlational design was selected because it helped to explain human behaviors or to predict likely outcomes. The methodology also views numbers to analyze the data using an objective rather than a subjective approach to support or refute a hypothesis being tested.

The qualitative and mixed-method methodologies was considered but not adopted for this study because of the sample size of participants from which to collect data, the number of known variables to collect to establish correlation, the selection of instruments to be used to collect data, and the short period of timeframe required to collect the data. The qualitative method uses unknown variables and the investigation into the research problem is based on the perspective and personal narratives of the participants. Unlike quantitative methods where the researcher explores and measures discreet variables to determine relationships and patterns, qualitative methods explore previously unexplored phenomena, and is useful for generating and testing a hypothesis. Qualitative research, however, is primarily used to understand patterns of thoughts and behaviors, and their meanings and inconsistencies (Kang, 2013).

In qualitative research, the researcher is centrally positioned which requires a degree of reflexivity. This privileged position creates an inherent power for potential bias, and ethical concerns between the researcher and its subjects. The quantitative and qualitative methodology, in spite of the similarities are both underpinned by positivist and Interpretivist understandings about the nature of their environment. Newman (2006) posits that quantitative researchers use a "positivist approach to social science" (p. 151). Most positivist researchers can collect measurable numeric data from study subjects using questionnaires or surveys to learn attitudes and beliefs, or opinions of study participants (Newman, 2006).

A quantitative approach was appropriate for this study because it involves testing the differences in relationships and examining the cause and effect connections between variables (LoBiondo-Wood & Harber, 2009). A quantitative numeric data can indicate the strength and direction of the association between variables. In a quantitative analysis, researchers can breakdown the numeric data obtained from the sample into parts to answer the research question enabling the researcher to describe trends, compare, relate or group variables of interest (Burns & Grove, 2003).

Research Design Appropriateness

The cross-sectional nature of this study was appropriate because it enables the researcher to select only a representative subset of the population to collect and analyze data, and to determine prevalence at a specific point in time. Using a cross-sectional design allowed the researcher to obtain the scores from multiple variables of interest to determine correlation from which the resulting correlation coefficient could indicate the degree of relationship among the variables. Experimental research, unlike cross-sectional research was not appropriate for this study because it requires the researcher to assign participants to control and treatment groups. Although the experimental research can establish causation and has higher internal validity because the participants are under the control of the researcher; however, observational studies have a greater external validity because it can establish association between variables within a scientific environment (Kang, 2013).

The use of a correlational design was appropriate for this study. A correlational design was appropriate because it determines the degree and direction of the relationship between the variables being explored. In this study, it was necessary to measure the variables (self-care management, self-care efficacy and self-care knowledge) at the same point in time in order to determine association, degree of the association and direction of the variables. Using correlations allowed the researcher to draw conclusions about the casual relationships between the variables (Salkind, 2012).

Population and Sampling Frame

The general population for this study are Black/African American women residing in the state of Texas. The specific population of interest in this study are middle-aged Black/African-American women (45 – 64 years of age) with Type II diabetes, residing in Dallas or Tarrant counties, north Texas, USA. According to the American Diabetes Association, a person has a diagnosis of Type II diabetes if s/he has a "fasting plasma glucose (FPG) level of 126 mg/dL (7.0 mmol/L) or higher, or a random plasma glucose of 200 mg/dL (11.1 mmol/L) or higher" (ADA, 2011, p.1).

The setting for this study was an online community in Dallas, Texas on the SurveyMonkey website specifically for residents of Dallas and Tarrant counties, north Texas. The survey instruments were posted on SurveyMonkey to allow residents of Dallas and Tarrant counties who met the eligibility criteria to participate in the study. Prospective participants were recruited using SurveyMonkey. This method of collecting data created anonymity so that the researcher may not interface with or directly observe the behavior of the participants.

According to the Texas Department of State Health Services (2015), as of 2013, an estimated 2,132,645 (10.9%) persons in the state have diagnosed diabetes. Among those, roughly 291,796 (13.3%) persons are African-Americans. It is not entirely clear how many middle-aged Black/African-American women have diabetes in Texas. Presently, it is estimated that 3.2 million Black/AfricanAmericans aged 20 years and older are affected by diabetes in the U.S. (ADA, 2013) and one in four Black/African-American woman aged 55 years and older has diabetes (ADA, 2013). It was this population that was the target for this study.

In a 2013 published study by the Texas Behavioral Risk Factor Surveillance System there is a higher prevalence of diabetes in Dallas and Tarrant counties, north Texas. The estimated population of persons living with diabetes in Tarrant county as of 2013 was 143,779 and 169,240 in Dallas county (THS, 2015). Although a survey of all middle-aged Black/African-American women with T2DM in north Texas may be ideal; however, the practice was not economically feasible giving the time and financial constraints involved. Therefore a sample of the population in Dallas and Tarrant counties was used for this study.

The sampling method that was used for this study was the convenience sampling method. The use of a non-probability convenience sampling technique was the preferred method of data collection for this study. Parahoo (1997) stated that in non-probability sampling, researchers can select the subjects that based on their judgement, have some knowledge of the phenomenon being studied. The purpose of sampling was to gather data about a subset of the population to make an inference that can be generalized to the population. According to Burns and Grove (2003), a large sample is required to obtain a confidence interval of 95%. To calculate the sample size needed for tests of one or two independent proportions, and for test of means, the power analysis "a priori" was used. The convenience sampling technique was used to select subjects for the study. Burns and Grove (2002) describe convenience sampling as "including subjects in the study because they happen to be in the right place at the right time" (p. 248).

The power analysis "a priori" was used to determine the sample size for this study. G*Power 3.1.9.2 is a statistical software program that is commonly used in behavioral, social and biomedical sciences (Faul, Erdfelder, Buchner, & Lang (2009). Faul et al. noted that power analysis measures the probability that a Type 2 error will not occur indicating the incidence of a false null hypothesis failing to be rejected. The correlation coefficient r or the regression coefficient R is the measure of effect size. Using Cohen's rule, a "small" effect size would be $d=0.2$, a "medium" effect size $d=0.5$, and a "large" effect size $d=0.8$. To determine the sample size for this study using G*Power 3.1.9.2, a sample size of 82 participants were obtained based on a medium effect size of ($d=0.3$), an alpha level of $a = .05$, and a power of 0.08 (Cohen, 1988). To compensate for possible incomplete surveys, the sample size was increased to 120. Figure 4. shows a G*power plot of the sample values calculated using a two-tailed test and a significance of $p=0.05$ and an effect size of 0.3 (Faul, Erdfelder, Buchner, & Lang, 2009).

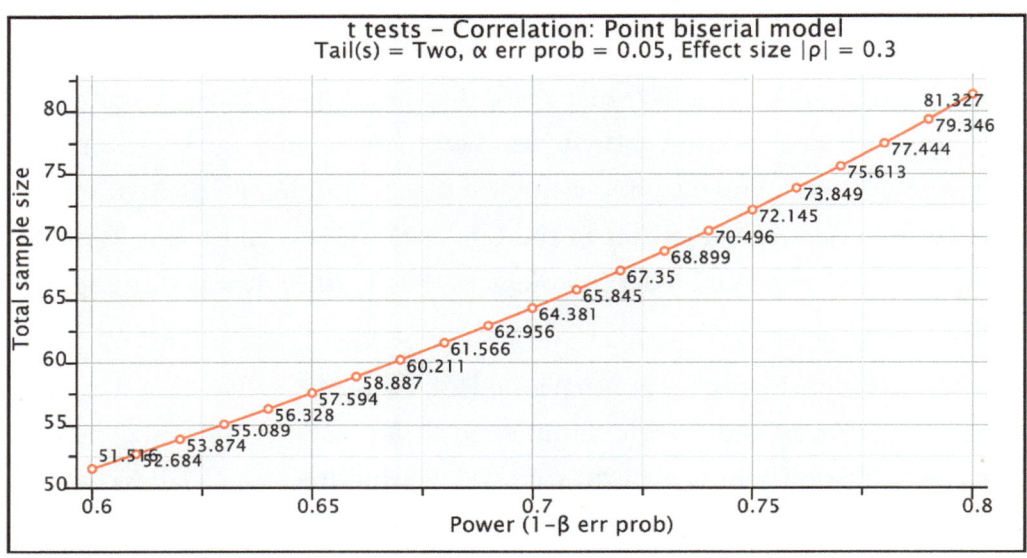

Figure 4. Plot of G*power for sample size selection (Faul et al., 2009)

Inclusion Criteria

The inclusion criteria was for participants to be: (a) Black/African American women, (b) self-report of being between the ages 45 and 64 years old at the time of recruitment into the study, (c) self-report of being diagnosed with T2DM and, (d) self-report of being a resident of Dallas or Tarrant county, north Texas. The only time the prospective participant was recruited to take the survey was if he or she met the inclusion criteria and consented to the study. Since the study was conducted in an online environment on SurveyMonkey platform, the researcher did not have any means of verifying or authenticating the validity of the demographic information provided by the prospective participant. Therefore, the researcher relied on the self-report provided by the prospective participant.

Informed Consent

In this study, the researcher did not have a face-to-face contact with the participants. Participants were required to use a computer to link to a SurveyMonkey site where the informed consent was posted. Participants were required to read and understand the informed consent and of their right to withdraw from the study without fear of retribution or loss of benefits. The participant were asked to answer "Yes" or "No" to "I have read and agree to the above Consent Agreement". A "Yes" signifies consent and the subject's agreement to participate in the study.

In this study, no personal identifiable information such as name, date of birth, social security number, hospital records, or home and work address was collected. The participants had a choice of completing the survey on the SurveyMonkey site or request a link to the survey at which point, an email address was required from participants in order to send them the link to take the survey at a later date. The IP tracking system on SurveyMonkey was turned off to avoid collecting personal identifiable information. Participants were not required to disclose any information outside the scope of the study. The demographic questionnaire and the survey instruments was posted on an electronic platform where participants can access and complete the survey at their convenience, 24/hrs a day.

If a participant elected to withdraw from the study, the participant was instructed to send an email to the researcher using the email address printed on the consent agreement informing him of her decision to withdraw from the study. All previously completed data were destroyed. The data collected from the active participants are sealed and kept in a safe under lock and key at the residence of the researcher for a minimum of three years, after which time the data will be shredded. Only the researcher have access to the data collected.

The Health and Human Services (HHS, 2014) has established human research guidelines and defined minimal risk as: "the probability and magnitude of harm or discomfort anticipated in the research are not greater in and of themselves than those ordinarily encountered in daily life or during the performance of routine physical or psychological examinations or tests" (p. 1). This study was a social science research that would not expose the subject to any physical harm. This study collected data in an online setting which did not require the researcher to interface with or directly communicate with the subject and as such, there was no foreseeable risk of physical or psychological harm to the participant.

However, since the study involved assessing psychosocial stressors with the subject, it is possible that the survey questions may have triggered emotional discomfort and cause anxieties which may have resulted in unanticipated harm to the participant. Prospective participants were encouraged to withdraw from the study if the subject encountered any emotional distress related to the study.

Confidentiality

Confidentiality of the information collected from this study was paramount to the researcher. Although no personal identifiable information such as names, addresses, telephone numbers, or other identifiable information was collected, the survey data is held in the strictest confidence and is placed under lock and key at the researcher's residence for three years after which it will be shredded and destroyed. Prior to the start of the study, to ensure anonymity the researcher disabled IP address tracking. This eliminated the names and IP addresses of the respondents from being collected and included in the survey results. Participants were assured that their information was confidential and would be destroyed after three years.

Geographic Location

The geographic location for this study was in Dallas and Tarrant counties, north Texas, United States.

Operational Definition of Variables and/or Constructs

Three variables were explored in this study: self-care efficacy, self-care knowledge, and self-care management. Self-care efficacy is the belief that an individual has the ability to create change by personal actions (Bandura, 1977). Operationally, self-care efficacy is determined by an individual's level of confidence to engage in diabetes management activities, such as blood glucose monitoring, engaging in diet and exercise, insulin administration, adhering to medication regimen, and responding to health challenges that may occur from time to time. This variable was measured on a categorical scale.

Self-care knowledge is the "facts, information, and skills acquired through experience or education; the theoretical or practical understanding of a subject" ("Knowledge,"2017). Operationally, self-care knowledge is a reasoned and reflective process. It refers to a patient's ability to acquire and use the information and skills through experience or education to facilitate performance of self-care. This variable was measured on a categorical scale.

Self-care management refers to a patient's ability to engage in the "daily activities that individuals undertake to keep their illness under control, minimize its impact on physical health status and functioning, and cope with the psychosocial sequelae of the illness" (Gallant, 2003, p. 170). Operationally, selfcare management in this context refers to "those activities individuals undertake in promoting their own health, preventing their own disease, limiting their own illness, and restoring their own health" (Levin, 1983, p. 1). This variable was measured on a categorical scale. The three variables are discussed in Chapter 2 under "Empirical Search on Variables".

Data Collection

The data collection process started following IRB approval. Prospective participants were recruited by distributing an advertising flyer (Appendix A) at public libraries, churches, community centers, picnic and church events, and at diabetes clinics such as the Joslin Diabetes Center, in the communities of Dallas and Tarrant counties. The advertising flyer provided a link to the study via a web link and a QR code that could be scanned with a smartphone. The researcher's email address and contact phone number were also printed on the advertising flyer should any prospective participant want to contact the researcher.

Prospective participants who met the criteria advertised in the flyer and wish to enroll in the study were required to use a computer or a smartphone to link to the advertising flyer online on the SurveyMonkey site. Upon agreeing that the participant met the criteria for the study, a link was sent directing them to the Consent Agreement. The participants were asked to answer "Yes" or "No" to "I have read and agree to the above Consent Agreement". A "Yes" signifies consent and the subject's agreement to participate in the study. A "No" signified not to consent to the study. If the participant elected not to consent to the study, the participant was disqualified and the link was closed.

The four survey instruments (Appendices C, D, E, & F) were consolidated into a single questionnaire used to collect data on the SurveyMonkey platform. The consolidation created continuity and made it convenient for the participant to respond to a single survey instrument rather than several instruments which could have potentially contributed to fatigue and lack of interest. During the survey, the participant could at any time stop and return to continue taking the rest of the survey without losing any data. However, the survey had to be completed within 30 days of the date of the informed consent. The process of collecting data continued until the sample size was exhausted, after which the survey was closed.

Data Storage and Preparation.

The data collected from SurveyMonkey was in machine readable form. After the data was collected, it was downloaded to a flash thumb drive to protect accidental erasure on SurveyMonkey database. The flash thumb drive was stored in a safe at the residence of the researcher. Subsequently, it was downloaded into an Excel sptreadsheet on the researcher's computer. The computer was password protected and stored safely at the resident of the researcher. No other user other than the researcher have access to the computer. Following the completion of the research study, the data was removed from the computer and stored on a flash thumb drive and then deleted from the computer. The researcher will destroy the flash thumb drive after three years following the completion of the study.

The data in the Excel spreadsheet was sanitized and subsequently uploaded into an SPSS database for data analysis. The sanitization process included: generating histograms of each variable to ensure it was not positively or negatively skewed with extreme values, coding raw data before transferring the data into a model, removing duplicate entries from the database, and removing extraneous characters and out-of-range data elements. The purpose of using a histogram was to graphically summarize the distribution of a univariate data set (Wilson, Voorhis, & Morgan, 2007).

Once data sanitization was completed, a scatter plot of each predictor variable was generated against the outcome variable to check for outliers. An outlier is "an observation that lies an abnormal distance from other values in a random sample from a population" (NIST, 2017, p. 1). Outliers are potentially erroneous information that could have been entered through data entry when the surveys were collected. If an outlier was identified, it was investigated and if necessary removed from the database. The scatter plot was checked for normality of the data to ensure the variables were normally distributed for continuous variables, and for homoscedasticity of the data.

Outliers are suspicious data points that could either be erroneous or extreme data. Although there are suggested scientific methods in dealing with outliers, the amount of data collected for this study may not lend itself to use a scientific method to determine whether the data should be removed or left to improve the "fit" of the regression line, if any, was generated. The method used was to examine each outlier independently for special properties, characteristics, or circumstances relevant to the outlier. For example, if age was reported as 99 years old when the target age was between 45 and 64, this was flagged as a data entry error. The approach was to examine the regression line, if any, with and without the outliers to determine their influence on the results. If the influence was substantial and it was determined that the data was not collected in error, then the researcher would present both analyses.

Instrumentation

In this study, data was collected for three variables - self-care efficacy, self-care knowledge, self-care management, and the demographic questionnaire using four survey instruments. The Demographic Questionnaire (Appendix C), the Diabetes Knowledge Test (Fitzgerald, Funnel, Anderson, Nwankwo, Stansfield, & Platt, 2016) to measure self-care knowledge (Appendix D), The Summary of Diabetes Self-Care Activities Scale (Toobert, Hampson, & Glasgow, 2000) to measure self-care management (Appendix E), and the Stanford Diabetes Self-care efficacy Scale (Stanford University, 2008) to measure self-care efficacy (Appendix F).

Demographic Questionnaire

The demographic questionnaire (Appendix C) is an 8-item self-survey designed to capture the participant's personal characteristics. The selected demographic data as shown on Appendix C are potentially moderators of the relationship between self-care efficacy, self-care knowledge, and self-care management. The demographic questionnaire asks information about race, types of medications used to treat diabetes, duration of illness, age-group, level of education, marital status, whether the patient had ever received diabetes education, and employment status. Some of the information contained in the questionnaire was used to test correlations with self-care knowledge, self-care efficacy, and self-care management. The demographic questionnaire instrument was created by the researcher.

Measure of the Summary of Diabetes Self-Care Activities Scale

The SDSCA (Appendix E) is an expanded 15-item, seven-point Likerttype scale which is a valid and reliable instrument used to assess levels of diabetes self-care behaviors across different components of the diabetes regimen (Toobert, Hampson, & Glasgow, 2000). The SDSCA questionnaire focuses on behaviorrelated patterns such as general diet and diabetes-specific diet (5-items), physical activity (2-items), foot care (5-items), blood-glucose testing (2-items), and medications (1-item) for people with diabetes. The instrument assesses the absolute frequency or consistency of diabetes self-care behaviors. Each subset of the scale is scored separately. For example, the instruments assess in the past 7 days, the number of days per week on which respondents engage in physical activities or the number of days in which a respondent ate five or more servings of fruits and vegetables. The instrument is self-administered in an adult population and takes about 15 to 20 minutes to complete. Table 2 illustrates the scoring of the SDSCA scale. Items in each subscale were summed up separately and the mean calculated.

Table 2. Scoring the SDSCA scale

Subscale	Mean (M) of Items	Items to Reverse Score
General Diet	1,2	
Specific Diet	3,4,5 with item 4 reversed	Reverse item 4 (0=7, 1=6, 2=5, 3=4, 4=3, 5=2, 6=1, 7=0).
Exercise	6,7	
Blood Glucose Testing	8,9	
Foot Care	10,11,12,13,14 with item 13 reversed	Reverse item 13 (0=7, 1=6, 2=5, 3=4, 4=3, 5=2, 6=1, 7=0).
Medications	15	

Research for this instrument was supported by the National Institutes of Health from 1983-2009. The validity of the instrument has been tested in several studies (see Table 3); one with three studies (Toobert & Glasgow, 1994), and one with seven studies (Toobert, Hampson, & Glasgow, 2000). The average reliability of the scale is .735. "A 2000 article in Diabetes Care provided normative data, inter-item and test-retest reliability, correlations between the SDSCA subscales and a range of criterion measures, and sensitivity to change from seven different studies" (Oregon Research Institute [ORI], 2012, p. 1). A written permission to use the SDSCA scale was obtained from the authors (see Appendix H).

Table 3. Cross-section of Studies that have used the SDSCA Scale

Study	Year	(n)	Type	Avg./Reliability
Bautista et al.	2016	331	Type II	0.62 (3 sub-scales)
Schmitt et al.	2016	430	Type I and II	0.686
Kim et al.	2015	90	Type II	0.791
Tol et al.	2012	140	Type II	0.77
Miller & Elasy	2008	131	Type II	0.81 (2 sub-scales)

Measure of the Diabetes Self-care Efficacy Questionnaire (DSEQ)

Self-care efficacy in this study was measured using the Stanford self-care efficacy scale. The DSEQ is an instrument used to measure diabetes self-care efficacy in people with diabetes. The scale is an 8-item Likert-type questionnaire used to measure the confidence of participants in performing diabetes self-care behaviors, including their ability to control diabetes, following a diet plan, eating meals every 4-5 hours, choosing the appropriate foods, increasing exercising regimen, closely monitoring blood glucose to avoid hyperglycemia or hypoglycemia, and determining when it is appropriate to visit a physician. Scores on the DSEQ is a linear scale ranging from 1 to 10, with 1 corresponding to "not at all confident" (low self-care efficacy) and 10 corresponding to "totally confident" (higher self-care efficacy). The total score is the mean (M) of all the scored items. The scale has been evaluated by many studies and shown to have an average internal consistency reliability of 0.828.

A review of the literature on the National Institutes of Health PUBMED database found that within the last five years, more than 834 research publications have cited the Stanford diabetes self-care efficacy scale to assess self-care efficacy in people with T2DM. Although most studies have used the instrument for longitudinal studies to compare baseline and follow-up results, researchers have used the instrument in cross-sectional studies of patients with T2DM. Based on search results from the NIH PUBMED database, more than 244 cross-sectional studies have used the Stanford diabetes self-care efficacy scale. Table 4 illustrates a cross-section of cross-sectional studies that have used and cited the Stanford diabetes self-care efficacy scale. No specific permission to use this instrument was required since the scale was available in the public domain (Appendix F).

Table 4. Cross-section of Studies that have used the Stanford Self-care efficacy scale

Study	Year	(n)	Type	Avg./Reliability
Shao, Yin, & Wan	2017	532	Type II	0.87
Carpenter et al.	2017	279	Glaucoma	0.86
Jacob et al.	2016	242	Type II	0.91
Kashani et al.	2016	119	Type II	0.89
Quinn et al.	2015	18	Type II	0.92
Huang, Zhao, Li, Jiang	2014	364	Type II	0.89
Liberman, Buckingham, Phillip	2014	334	Type I and II	0.88
Loeb, Steffensmeier, Kassab	2012	131	Self-rated Health Status	0.92

Huang, Zhao, Li, and Jiang (2014) used the Stanford self-care efficacy scale to explore the factors influencing diabetes self-management behavior among 364 Chinese patients in Chengdu city, Western China. The researchers used several instruments to collect data. Diabetes self-care efficacy was measured using the Stanford self-care efficacy scale with internal consistency reliability of 0.9. Diabetes knowledge was assessed using the KAP (knowledge-AttitudePractice) theory. The instrument had a content validity ratio (CVR) of 0.965 and for each dimension; the CVR was 0.900-1. Self-management beliefs were measured using a diabetes-specific scale developed on the basis of the Health Belief model (HBM). The content validity of the scale was 0.81, the test-retest reliability was 0.78 – 0.82, and the Cronbach's alpha was 0.79.

Measure of Diabetes Knowledge Test (DKT)

The Diabetes Knowledge Test (Appendix D) was adapted from the Michigan Diabetes Knowledge Scale which was developed by researchers at the Michigan Diabetes Research and Training Center. The scale is a 23-item multiplechoice questionnaire to assess patient's diabetes-related knowledge including medication taking, blood glucose control, diet and exercise, and complications. The instrument has a subscale of 14 items that is appropriate for patients with T1DM and T2DM, and a subscale of 9 additional items for assessing insulin knowledge that is appropriate for both T1DM and T2DM using insulin therapy. The readability of the scale was measured using the Flesch-Kincaid grade level. The scale can be read at the 6th grade level. The internal reliability of the scale is 0.61, the Chronbach's ranged from 0.69 to 0.71, and the item correlation with total knowledge score ranged between 0.23 and 0.45 (Fitzgerald et al., 2016). No specific permission to use this instrument was required since the scale was available in the public domain. The DKT was reproduced courtesy of the Michigan Diabetes Research Center (MDRC).

The DKT instrument is used by students, researchers, and clinicians to assess a patient's overall knowledge of diabetes. The instrument consists of two sections: the general section consists of 14 items (items 1 – 14) which is appropriate for all patients with diabetes. The second section consists of 9 items (items 15 – 23) which is appropriate for people with diabetes using insulin. The instrument was scored by adding individual scale items and arriving at a total score and calculating the mean and standard deviation of the scores. Each correct item scores one point for a total of 23 points. Lower scores indicated poor knowledge of diabetes. Conversely, higher scores indicated better knowledge of diabetes.

Data Analysis

Data analysis for this study was performed using descriptive, inferential, correlation analysis, and multiple logistics regression statistics. The statistical method used was a two-tailed test and the hypothesis was tested at the .05 level of significance.

Descriptive Statistics

Descriptive statistics was used to describe the demographic data. The demographic data was analyzed according to level of measurement of the data. Frequencies and percentages were used for nominal and ordinal data. Measures of central tendency, measures of dispersion, and frequencies were used to analyze the interval and ratio level variables.

The distribution of scores on the research instruments were inspected for normalcy. Normal distribution of scores is needed to test a hypothesis using correlational statistics. The descriptive statistics that was used for the variables are median, mode, counts, and percentage calculations. A histogram and bar graphs were generated to visualize and describe the data since the data is non-parametric.

Inferential Statistics

Inferential statistics was used to make inferences from the data collected. Pearson correlation coefficients was used to explore inter-relationships among the variables of self-care efficacy, self-care knowledge, and self-care management after testing the data for normality and linearity between the variables, and homoscedasticity of the data. The hypothesis in this study was tested using multiple correlation analysis. Since there are more than two variables to be explored in this study, correlation analysis is appropriate to explore and describe the relationships between the variables (Burnes & Grove, 2001). The variables (self-care efficacy, self-care knowledge, and self-care management) in the multivariate correlation model will all be measured on a categorical scale since all the data is ordinal (Cohen, 1988). The objective of this study is not to determine causation or predict the variance in the value of the variables but to understand the correlation between self-care efficacy, self-care knowledge, and self-care maintenance in middle-aged Black/African-American women with T2DM in north Texas.

Correlation Analysis

The purpose of using correlation analysis in this correlational study is to predict scores and explain the relationship among the variables. In correlation research designs, the researcher uses correlation statistics to describe and measure the degree and direction of the relationship between two or more variables of interest. Correlations between variables measures the strength of the relationships and how well the variables are related. Correlation is simply a measure of the magnitude of the association between variables. It does not assume that there is a dependent and independent variable among the two.

Three types of correlations were considered in this study: Pearson Coefficient (r), Spearman's rho coefficient (r), and Kendall's tau. Unlike the Pearson's r, which is a parametric test and expects normality in the distribution of the data, the Spearman rank order correlation is a non-parametric test. It was selected over the other correlation methods because of: a) its ability to measure variables that have non-linear tendency, b) the measurement level of the data is ordinal, c) it is most suitable for variables with non-normal distribution or highly skewed data, and d) it is a suitable alternative to Pearson's r for measuring non- parametric data.

In comparison to Pearson's r which indicates the linear relationships between two variables, Spearman rank order measures the strength of the monotone association between two ordinal variables. According to Hauke and Kossowski (2011) Spearman's correlation coefficient "assesses how well an arbitrary monotonic function can describe the relationship between two variables, without making any assumptions about the frequency distribution of the variables" (p. 89). As with Pearson's r, the Spearman rank order correlation can range in values from -1 to +1. As the correlation coefficient reaches 0 (zero), it indicates that there is no relationship between the variables (Salkind, 2012). According to Cohen (1988), the correlation coefficients for r, rho, or tau are .10 to .29 (small association between the variables), 0.30

to 0.49 (moderate association), and 0.50 and above (significant or large associations). A histogram was generated to visually determine the normality of the data for non-categorical variables, if any.

A bivariate data analysis was performed on the data. Bivariate Data Analysis is a statistical technique used to analyze data arising from two or more variables. Other statistical tests that were performed on the data includes the Pearson's Chi Square Test and the Mann-Whitney U-Tests. The Mann-Whitney U-Test is a statistical test used to compare differences between two independent groups when the data is not normally distributed. The test can be used to determine the strength of the monotone association between the score on self-care knowledge and the highest level of education attained by the participant. The Mann Whitney U-Test is the non-parametric alternative to the independent t-test.

The Pearson's Chi Square test (χ^2) is designed to analyze categorical data. It is a test of independence. The test is used to evaluate whether two variables are independent or related. It does not provide any inferences about causation. Table 5 summarizes the statistical approach to data analysis that was performed on each variable and the scales used to collect the data (Salkind, 2012).

Table 5. Statistical Approach to Data Analysis

Research Related Questions	Null Hypothesis	Scales/Survey Items	Statistical Data Type	Approach
RQ# 1 – What is the relationship, if any, between self-care efficacy and self-care knowledge in middle-aged Black/ AfricanAmerican women in north Texas with T2DM?	There is no statistically significant relationship between self-care efficacy and selfcare knowledge in middle-aged Black/African-American women in north Texas with T2DM	Demographic Questionnaire; Stanford Diabetes Self- care efficacy Scale; Diabetes Knowledge Test	Categorical level Ordinal variables	Kendall's tau, Bivariate Analysis, Pearson's Chi square test, ANOVA, Binary logistic regression
RQ# 2 – What is the relationship, if any, between self-care efficacy and self-care management in middle-aged Black/ AfricanAmerican women in north Texas with T2DM?	There is no statistically significant relationship between self-care efficacy and selfcare management in middle-aged Black/African-American women in north Texas with T2DM.	Demographic Questionnaire; level, Diabetes Self- care efficacy Scale; Summary of Diabetes Selfcare Activities Scale	Categorical level Ordinal variables	Kendall's tau, Bivariate Analysis, Pearson's Chi square test, ANOVA, Binary logistic regression

Research Related Null Scales/Survey Statistical Questions Hypothesis Items Data Type Approach				
RQ# 3 – What is the relationship, if any, between self-care knowledge and self-care management in middle-aged Black/African-American women in north Texas with T2DM?	There is no statistically significant relationship between self-care knowledge and self-care management in middle-aged Black/African-American women in north Texas with T2DM	Demographic Questionnaire; Diabetes Knowledge Test; Summary of Diabetes Selfcare Activities Scale	Categorical level, Ordinal variables	Kendall's tau, Bivariate Analysis, Pearson's Chi square test, ANOVA, Binary logistic regression.

Validity and Reliability

Validity.

Validity refers to a measure of the actual instrument it is purported to measure. Several types of validity measurements exist: face validity, internal and external validity, criterion-related validity, sampling validity, and formative validity.

Internal Validity. Internal validity refers to the degree to which the results are attributable to the independent variable and not some other rival explanation. Internal validity can be affected by the type of research design or by several potential threats including testing effects and instrumentation. Internal validity encompasses analyzing random and systematic error. Random error in instrumentation is an error that is caused by unknown and unpredictable changes in either the instrument itself or in environmental conditions. Random error is pervasive in all measuring instruments and testing samples. It cannot be eliminated; however, it can be "minimized by increasing the sample size (Tripepi et al., 2008, p. 148). The random error in this study is minimized by the selection of instruments that have been validated by many studies in the field of diabetes and health research. Systematic error (bias) refers to the tendency to consistently underestimate or overestimate a true value. The systematic error can occur as a result of sampling bias.

External Validity. External Validity refers to the generalization of the hypothesized relationships across settings, persons, and times. The two primary sources of external validity was reviewed: (a) Interaction of selection and (b) reactive effects of testing.

Interaction of selection. The study was specifically limited to the north Texas area (Dallas and Tarrant counties) and to Black/African American women populations only, and cannot be generalized to larger populations.

Reactive effects of testing. The subjects in this study knew that he or she was participating in an online survey and that their responses were being monitored by the researcher. As a result, the subjects may experience the novelty of participating in the research, which researchers refer to as the Hawthorne Effect. The Hawthorne Effect is the "consequent awareness of being studied, and possible impact on behavior" (McCambridge, Witton, & Elbourne, 2014, p. 1)

Threats to validity. Threats to validity refers to any uncontrolled extraneous variables or circumstances that may affect the outcome of a study. In this study, the two threats to internal validity were selection bias and testing instruments used to collect data. Alexander, Lopes, Ricchetti-Masterson, and Yeatts (2013) noted that selection bias can occur in research when improper procedures are used by investigators for selecting a sample population. The threat to external validity of this study refers to the generalizability of the study to the general population. The use of a non-probability convenience sampling method limited the generalization of this study to the public. Another significant threat to the external validity of this study was the setting to be studied. This study was specifically designed to survey middle-aged Black/African American women residing in Dallas or Tarrant County, north Texas using SurveyMonkey. Due to the anonymity and limitation of IP tracking being disabled for this study, the researcher may not have been able to distinguish subjects who may participate in the survey from other geographical settings purporting to be residents of Dallas or Tarrant counties, north Texas.

Reliability

Reliability refers to the degree to which an instrument produces consistent results. Several types of reliability and validity measurements exist: test-retest reliability, inter-rater reliability, and internal consistency reliability; face validity, criterion-related validity, sampling validity, and formative validity). Nunnaly (1978) has suggested 0.7 to be an acceptable reliability coefficient but lower thresholds have sometimes been used in the literature. One of the most popular reliability statistics used in social science research is the Cronbach's alpha (Cronbach, 1951). This statistic determines the internal consistency or average correlation of items in a survey instrument to gauge its reliability and it has been accepted by most researchers in social science research as a rule of thumb for average correlations. The reliability of each instrument in this study (Self-care efficacy Scale for Diabetes, Diabetes Knowledge Test, and Summary of Diabetes Self-Care Activities Scale) were all tested by their respective authors and are reported under the appropriate headings in the previous sections (Cronbach, 1971).

The reliability and validity of the DKT were supported in both samples. Cronbach's coefficient alpha was used to calculate reliability separately for each sample and for both samples combined. The Cronbach's coefficient alpha for the general test for the community, MDPH, and total was 0.70, 0.71, and 0.71, respectively, and for insulin use was 0.74, 0.76, and 0.75, respectively. Therefore, the coefficient alpha values for the general test and the insulin-use subscale indicated that both were reliable ($\alpha > .70$). The reliability estimates for the two samples were similar. In the current study, alpha reliabilities for the knowledge general test, the insulin-use subscale, and for the total DKT were: .32, .25, and .49 respectively (Fitzgerald et al., 2016).

Summary

This chapter described the study design and methodology used. The descriptive, quantitative, non-experimental research with a correlation design was proposed for this study. Cross sectional surveys enable researchers to observe many subjects at the same point in time. The scales used in this study were all standardized and revealed high reliability and validity measures. Data analysis included Kendall's tau, Mann Whitney U-Test, and Pearson's Chi Square test. A convenience and snowball sampling method and sample size were recognized as limitations; however, findings from this study were not generalizable but might still help support or refute earlier studies on the topic.

The descriptive nature of the study enabled the researcher to describe the association between the variables and within groups. The descriptive nature also enabled the researcher to gather and organize the data, and to tabulate the results, and provide a summary of the findings including an explanation of the magnitude and correlation between the variables. In contrast with the Pearson's correlation which was used specifically for data that is normally distributed, Kendall's tau was more appropriate for this type of study because of its ability to measure nonnormal distributed or highly skewed data.

CHAPTER 4

Results

The purpose of this descriptive, quantitative, correlational study was to assess the association and magnitude of the relationship, if any, between diabetesrelated knowledge, self-care efficacy, and self-care management in middle-aged Black/African-American women (45 – 64 years of age) with T2DM in north Texas. Chapter 3 presented the research methodology, research approach, research design including population and samples, instrumentation and operationalization of constructs, data collection procedures, plan for data analysis, threats to validity, and ethical concerns. The study's three hypothesis were tested and the findings and results including data analysis is presented in this chapter.

Research Design and Methods

A descriptive correlational research design was selected to examine the relationship between the variables self-care knowledge, self-care efficacy, and self-care management. To address the research questions, a quantitative descriptive method with a correlational design was selected to examine the relationship between the variables. Since a correlation does not establish causation, a bivariate correlation study was conducted using Kendall's tau in order to examine the association between the variables.

Research Questions and Hypothesis

Three research questions were asked in this study.

RQ# 1 – What is the relationship, if any, between self-care efficacy and self-care knowledge in middle-aged Black/African-American women with T2DM, in north Texas?

RQ# 2 – What is the relationship, if any, between self-care efficacy and self-care management in middle-aged Black/African-American women with T2DM, in north Texas?

RQ# 3 – What is the relationship, if any, between self-care knowledge and self-care management in middle-aged Black/African-American women with T2DM, in north Texas?

Population and Sampling

The general population for this study was Black/African American women living in Texas. The target population was middle-aged Black/African American women (45 to 64 years of age), living in Dallas or Tarrant County, Texas with T2DM. A sample size of 82 participants were obtained using the G*Power 3.1.9.2, based on a medium effect size of (d=0.3), an alpha level of $a = .05$, and a power of 0.08 (Cohen, 1988). However, 129 participants responded to the advertising flyer. Of the 129, only 120 completed the survey on SurveyMonkey®. All study participants who completed the survey met all four criteria for the study: Black/African American female, at least 18 years or older, had T2DM, and lived in Dallas county or Tarrant county, Texas.

Data Collection

The data collection process started following approval from the University of Phoenix IRB. Participants were recruited via flyers posted at churches, diabetes clinics, and at public libraries. The target population was middle-aged Black/African American women with T2DM in Dallas and Tarrant County, Texas. Data was collected using non-probability convenience sampling. The online survey was hosted on SurveyMonkey®. Informed consent was obtained in electronic form before the prospective participants could proceed with the survey.

The survey data was collected using four instruments: the Demographic questionnaire (Appendix C), Diabetes Knowledge Test (Appendix D), The Summary of Diabetes Self-care Activities Scale (Appendix E), and the Stanford Diabetes Self-care efficacy Scale (Appendix F). The four instruments were combined into a single scale on SurveyMonkey® consisting of 53 questions to ease continuity in taking the survey. A link to the survey was sent to participants who responded to the advertising flyer. Data collection was stopped once the number of surveys reached 129. The data collected from SurveyMonkey® were downloaded into Microsoft Excel 2010 database for sanitization before it was uploaded into SPSS version 25 (IBM Corp., Armonk, NY, USA) for data analysis. In Excel, a histogram of the data for each variable was generated to check for the summary distribution of a univariate data set (Wilson, Voorhis, & Morgan, 2007).

Descriptive Statistics.

This research was a descriptive, quantitative study, with a correlational design. Descriptive statistics were employed and used to calculate measures of central tendency to summarize information about the variables and to describe the data. Standard deviations were calculated to interpret the distribution of the data. The sample included ($N = 120$) participants. All participants self-identified as middle-aged (45 - 64 years of age), Black/African American female with Type II diabetes, and residing in either Dallas or Tarrant County, north Texas. Table 6 illustrates the demographic characteristics of the participants.

Table 6. Demographic Characteristics of the Participants

Demographics	n	%
Medication type:		
Insulin and Medications	40	33.3
Insulin only	6	5.0
Medications only	74	61.7
Duration of illness:		
1 – 4 years	20	16.7
5 – 10 years	52	43.3
11 – 15 years	32	26.7
Over 15 years	16	13.3
Age group:		
Under 18 years	0	
18 – 24 years	0	
25 – 34 years	0	
35 – 44 years	0	
45 – 54 years	81	67.5
55 – 64 years	39	32.5
Level of education:		
Did not attend school	0	
Some high school	0	
Graduated from high school	7	5.8
Some college	29	24.2
Graduated from college	50	41.7

Demographics	*n*	%
Some graduate school	18	15.0
Completed graduate school	16	13.3
Marital status:		
Single	58	48.3
Married	62	51.7
Diabetes education:		
No	67	55.8
Yes	53	44.2
Employment status:		
Employed, working full time	66	55.0
Employed, working part-time	34	28.3
Not employed	14	11.7
Retired	2	1.7
Disabled, not able to work	4	3.3

Table 7 depicts a descriptive statistic for self-care knowledge, self-care management, and self-care efficacy. As shown in the table, 75.65% is the mean percentage of correct answers for self-care knowledge, with a mean of 17.4±2.056, and interquartile range of 9, indicating a high degree of diabetes knowledge among the sample. Similarly, the mean percentage of correct answers for self-care management and self-care efficacy are 74.84% and 53.45% respectively. For self-care knowledge, the median was 17.5 out of 23 (76.00%). However, no participant was able to score 23 points. Only 6 (5%) participants out of 120 scored above 20 points, indicating a significant gap in diabetes knowledge among this cohort. The median for self-care management was 85 out of 105 (80.95%) indicating a high degree of self-care knowledge. The results show that only 4 (3%) of the sample managed to score over 102 points indicating that the average respondent performed self-care management activities less than 7 days a week as recommended for self-care activities. The median for self-care efficacy was 43 out of 80 (53.75%) indicating moderate self-care efficacy to carry out selfcare activities.

Table 7. Descriptive statistics for Self-care Knowledge, Self-care Management and Self-care Efficacy

Variable	*n*	Mean	±SD	Median	IR[1]	Mean % of correct answers
Self-care knowledge	120	17.4	2.056	17.5	9	75.65
[1]IR = Interquartile Range						

Variable	n	Mean	±SD	Median	IR1	Mean % of correct answers
Self-care management	120	78.58	17.986	85.0	58	74.84
Self-care efficacy	120	42.76	7.899	43.0	34	53.45
[1]IR = Interquartile Range						

Inferential Statistics

Bivariate statistics was used to determine statistical relationship between the variables. Specifically, Kendall's tau correlation coefficient was used to determine the strength and direction of the correlation coefficient between the variables. Pearson chi-square tests were performed to determine significance of the relationship between the variables. Mann-Whitney U-tests were performed on the demographic variables: medication type, duration of illness, age, level of education, marital status, diabetes education, and employment status. All statistical tests conducted were two-tailed and a p-value < 0.05 was considered significant resulting in the rejection of the null hypothesis. Table 8 depicts a bivariate correlation between diabetes education, and the variables self-care knowledge, self-care management, and self-care efficacy. The findings show that diabetes education was significantly correlated with self-care knowledge (p < .001), self-care management (p < .001), and self-care efficacy (p < .001).

Table 8. Bivariate Correlations between Diabetes Education, and
Self-care Knowledge, Management, and Efficacy

Bivariate Correlations					
		Diabetes	Self-care	Self-care	Self-care
Diabetes education	Correlation Coefficient	1.000	.352**	.679**	.547**
	Sig. (2-tailed)	.	.000	.000	.000
	N	120	120	120	120
Self-care knowledge	Correlation Coefficient	.352**	1.000	.172**	.275**
	Sig. (2-tailed)	.000	.	.009	.000
	N	120	120	120	120
Self-care management	Correlation Coefficient	.679**	.172**	1.000	.370**
	Sig. (2-tailed)	.000	.009	.	.000
	N	120	120	120	120
(Kendall's tau b) education knowledge management efficacy					
**. Correlation is significant at the 0.01 level (2-tailed).					

Bivariate Correlations					
Self-care efficacy	Correlation Coefficient	.547**	.275**	.370**	1.000
	Sig. (2-tailed)	.000	.000	.000	.
	N	120	120	120	120
(Kendall's tau b) education knowledge management efficacy					
**. Correlation is significant at the 0.01 level (2-tailed).					

Self-care Knowledge

Self-care knowledge was obtained from the DKT (Appendix D) scale. The scores were divided into two subsections: a general subscale pertaining to general knowledge of diabetes (Items 1 to 14), and an insulin only subscale (Items 15 – 23) for patients who use insulin to manage their diabetes. Each question had three or four multiple choice answers. Each correct answer choice scored one point, and each incorrect answer choice scored zero points.

The scores on the DKT were not categorized; therefore, three standard categories were created for the General DKT test: 1 to 6 (Low), 7 to 11 (Average), 12 to 14 (High). The insulin subscale (15 to 23) was included in the overall combined score. However, non-insulin participants were not expected to score high since some did not have comprehensive knowledge of insulin use. The combined scores were added and the mean calculated. The maximum score was 23 points. A higher score on the general subscale indicated higher knowledge of general diabetes symptoms. Conversely, a lower score on the general subscale indicated less knowledge of diabetes symptoms.

Table 9 illustrates the descriptive statistics of the self-care knowledge obtained from the DKT Questionnaire. There were no combined knowledge scores below 12 points. Roughly 17.5% of respondents had an average knowledge score of 11 points or below and 82.5% had high knowledge of diabetes. When the general score was combined with the insulin knowledge score, only 2 (1.66%) respondents using combined insulin and medications (pills) scored above 20 points. Combining the two scores (general knowledge and insulin knowledge) resulted in a mean score of (17.40±2.056) for the two categories.

Table 9. Descriptive Statistics of Self-care Knowledge

		Low knowledge (Items 1 - 6)	Average knowledge (7 - 11)	High knowledge (12 - 14)	Insulin knowledge (15 - 23)	Combined knowledge (1 - 23)
		Self-care Knowledge Statistics				
N	Valid	120	120	120	120	120
	% Score	0%	17.5%	82.5%		
Mean		5.61	10.14	12.99	4.41	17.40
Median		6.00	11.00	14.00	5.00	17.50
Std. Deviation		.677	1.197	1.338	1.481	2.056
Range		3	4	4	8	9
Minimum		3	7	10	0	12
Maximum		6	11	14	8	21

Self-care knowledge was inversely correlated with Medication Type ($r = 0.575$, $p < 0.001$). The DKT was administered to three groups of participants using combined diabetes medications (pills) and insulin, insulin only, and medications (pills) only. The results show that 74 (61.7%) used medications (pills) only, 6 (5%) used insulin only, and 40 (33.3%) used a combination of insulin and medications (pills). Participants using insulin only 6 (27.3%) and combined medication and insulin 16 (72.7%) had greater self-care knowledge of diabetes. The chi-square test of independence showed a statistically strong evidence of a relationship between Medication Type and self-care knowledge, $X^2 (20, 120) = 107.804$, $p < .001$. An analysis of variance found no significant differences in self-care knowledge across groups that use insulin and medications, insulin only, and medications only, $F (2,117) = 0.576$, $p = .564$.

Self-care knowledge was significantly associated with Diabetes education ($r = 0.352$, $p < 0.001$). Diabetes Education was dichotomized as received or did not receive diabetes education ("Y/N"). Roughly 53 (44.2%) indicated receiving diabetes education compared with 67 (55.8%) who did not indicate receiving diabetes education classes. Twelve (22.6%) participants who received diabetes education and 10 (45.5%) participants who did not receive diabetes education had higher self-care knowledge. The chi-square test of independence showed a statistically strong evidence of a relationship between Diabetes education and self-care knowledge, $X^2 (10, 120) = 29.958$, $p = 0.001$. An analysis of variance found significant differences in self-care knowledge across the groups that had received diabetes education and those that did not receive diabetes education, $F (1,118) = 11.816$, $p = .001$.

Self-care knowledge was significantly associated with Duration of illness ($r = 0.690$, $p < 0.001$). Fifty two (43.3%) participants had diabetes between 5 to 10 years, 32 (26.7%) had diabetes between 11 to 15 years, and 16 (13.3%) had diabetes over 15 years. However, 72.7% with diabetes over 15 years demonstrated more self-care knowledge compared to 27.3% with diabetes between 11 to 15 years. The results of a chi-square test of independence showed a statistically strong evidence of a relationship between duration of illness and self-care knowledge, $X^2 (30, 120) = 194.899$, $p < .001$, indicating that people who had longer symptoms of the disease had greater self-care knowledge. An analysis of variance found significant differences in self-care knowledge across the four duration of illnesses groups, $F (3,116) = 9.370$, $p = .000$.

Self-care knowledge was significantly associated with Age ($r = 0.383$, $p < 0.001$). Individuals below 45 years or above 64 years old were excluded from participating in the study. Roughly 67.5% of the sample were 45 – 54 years of age. The results showed 18 (81.8%) participants (55 – 64 years of age) had significant more self-care knowledge compared to 4 (18.2%) participants (45 – 54 years of age). The chi-square test of independence showed a statistically strong evidence of a relationship between Age and self-care knowledge, $X^2 (10, 120) = 35.9$, $p < .001$, indicating that participants over the age of 54 years had more self-care knowledge of diabetes. An analysis of variance found significant differences in self-care knowledge across the two age groups, $F (1,119) = 8.244$, $p = .005$.

Self-care knowledge was significantly associated with Education ($r = 0.226$, $p = 0.001$). Fifty (41.7%) graduated from college, 29 (24.2%) received some college education, 18 (15%) received some graduate school, 16 (13.3%) completed graduate school, and 7 (5.8%) graduated from high school. However, post-graduate knowledge did not significantly contribute to self-care knowledge. Only 8 (36.4%) participants with higher self-care knowledge were college graduates compared to 5 (27.8%) participants with some graduate school, and 4 (18.2%) with graduate degrees. The results of a chi-square test of independence showed a statistically strong evidence of a relationship between Education and self-care knowledge, $X^2 (40, 120) = 80.432$, $p < .001$. 1.585). An analysis of variance found significant differences in self-care knowledge across the levels of education, $F (4,115) = 3.254$, $p = .014$.

Self-care knowledge was not significantly associated with marital status ($r = 0.093$, $p = 0.231$). Marital status was dichotomized as single or married. Sixty two (51.7%) participants were married compared to 58 (48.3%) single participants. Fourteen (22.6%) participants who were reported as married had significantly higher scores in the knowledge test compared with 8 (36.4%) of single participants. The results of a chi-square test of independence did not show a statistically strong evidence of a relationship between Marital status and self-care knowledge, $X^2 (10, 120) = 9.224$, $p = 0.511$. An analysis of variance found no significant differences in self-care knowledge across the two marital status groups, $F (1,118) = 0.113$, $p = .737$.

Self-care knowledge was not significantly associated with Employment status ($r = 0.104$, $p = 0.887$). Sixty six (55.0%) participants were employed and working full time, 34 (28.3%) were employed and working part-time, 14 (11.7%) were not employed, 2 (1.7%) were retired, and 4 (3.3%) were disabled. The results of a chi-square test of independence did not show a statistically strong evidence of a relationship between Employment status and self-care knowledge, $X^2 (40, 120) = 29.578$, $p = 0.130$. An analysis of variance found no significant differences in self-care knowledge across employment groups, $F (4,115) = 0.794$, $p = .531$.

Cronbach's alpha was calculated on the percentage of correct answers for the combined subscales (general test and insulin subscales) and showed an alpha reliability scale of 0.77. The Cronbach's alpha for the general test subscale was 0.84 and 0.78 for the insulin use subscale, using a sample of ($N= 120$). The reliability of both subscales were consistent with the findings in the literature (Fitzgerald et al., 2016). Figure 5 below represents the histogram of self-care knowledge scores. As shown in the histogram, most of the scores are skewed to the right of the mean (17.4±2.056) and a long left tail of the data, indicating a high degree of self-care knowledge among the sample.

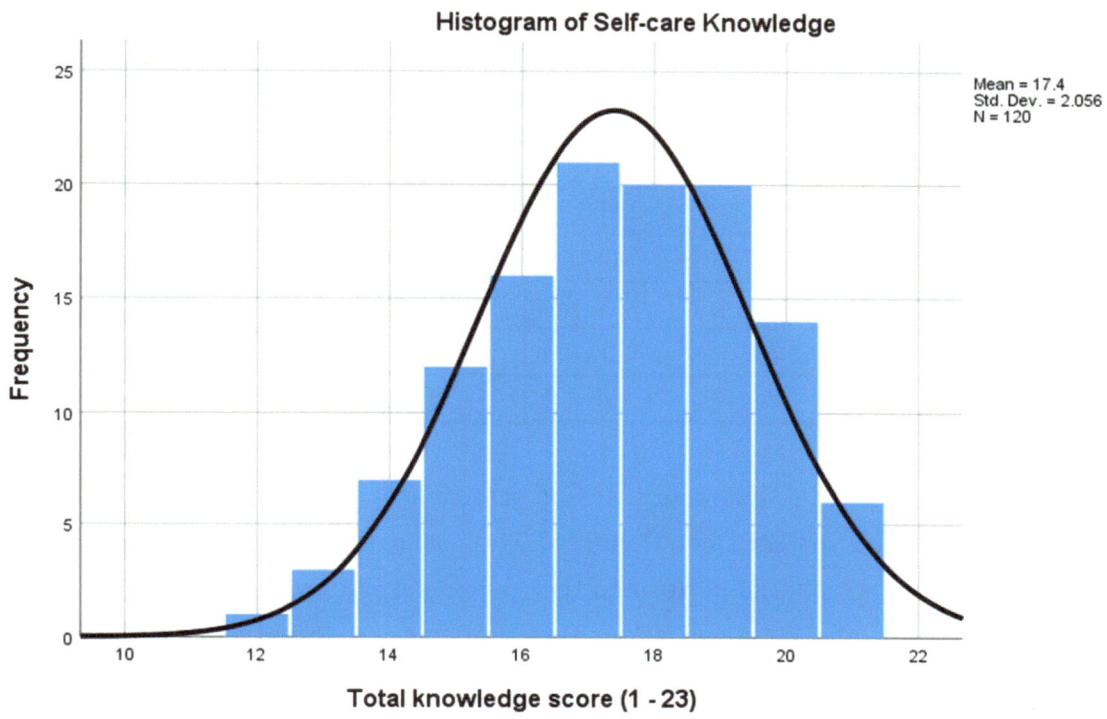

Figure 5. Histogram of Self-care Knowledge Scores

Self-care Management

Self-care management was measured using the SDSCA scale, an expanded 15-item, seven-point Likert scale used to assess self-management behavior of individuals with diabetes in the past 7 days. Each item on the scale scores 7 points for a maximum score of 105 points. Table 10 depicts the descriptive statistics of the self-care management obtained from the SDSCA scale. Self-care management behaviors were categorized into: diet, physical activity, blood glucose testing, foot care, and medications. The highest self-care management score (103) was obtained by 4 (3.33%) of the sample and the lowest self-care management score (45) was obtained by 3 (2.5%). Roughly 47 (39.16%) of the sample scored above the mean (78.58±17.986) indicating that less participants engaged in self-care behaviors.

Table 10. Descriptive Statistics of Self-care Management

Self-care Management Statistics							
		Diet	Physical Activity	Blood Glucose Testing	Foot Care	Medications	Combined Self-care Behaviors
N	Valid	120	120	120	120	120	120
	Missing	0	0	0	0	0	0
Mean		27.24	10.51	10.43	25.28	5.13	78.58
Median		28.50	11.50	11.00	27.00	6.00	85.00
Std. Deviation		6.503	3.373	3.078	6.775	1.771	17.986
Range		24	14	12	25	7	58
Minimum		11	0	2	10	0	45
Maximum		35	14	14	35	7	103

Table 11 depicts the demographic characteristics of participants who followed their self-care management behaviors in the last SEVEN Days. Roughly 50 (41.7%) participants followed their eating plan in the last SEVEN DAYS, 41 (34.2%) performed their blood sugar test daily in the last SEVEN DAYS, while 31 (25.8%) took their diabetes medications as recommended daily in the last SEVEN DAYS. The Cronbach's alpha for this test (.084) is consistent with other studies in the literature.

Table 11. Characteristics of Respondents Who Correctly Engaged in Self-care Behaviors

	Question	n	%[1]
1	On how many of the last SEVEN DAYS have you followed your eating plan	50	41.7
2	On Average, over the past month, how many DAYS PER WEEK have you followed your eating plan?	48	40.0
3	On how many of the last SEVEN DAYS did you eat five or more servings of fruits and vegetables	49	40.8
4	On how many of the last SEVEN DAYS did you eat high fat foods such as red meat or full-at dairy products?	49	40.8

	Question	n	% [1]
5	On how many of the last SEVEN DAYS did you space carbohydrates evenly through the day?	35	29.2
6	On how many of the last SEVEN DAYS did you participate in at least 30 minutes of physical activity? *(Total minutes of continuous activity, including walking).*	43	35.8
7	On how many of the last SEVEN DAYS did you participate in a specific exercise session (such as such swimming, walking, biking) other than what you do around the house or as part of your work?	36	30.0
8	On how many of the last SEVEN DAYS did you test your blood sugar?	41	34.2
9	On how many of the last SEVEN DAYS did you test your blood sugar the number of times recommended by your health care provider?	38	31.7
10	On how many of the last SEVEN DAYS did you check your feet?	43	35.8
11	On how many of the last SEVEN DAYS did you inspect the inside of your shoes?	40	33.3
12	On how many of the last SEVEN DAYS did you wash your feet?	31	25.8
13	On how many of the last SEVEN DAYS did you soak your feet?	36	30.0
14	On how many of the last SEVEN DAYS did you dry between your toes after washing?	35	29.2
15	On how many of the last SEVEN DAYS did you take your recommended diabetes medication	31	25.8

Table 12 depicts the correlation table between self-care management and the demographic variables. As shown, there is a moderate correlation between selfcare management and duration of illness ($r = 0.146$, $p < .05$), age ($r = 0.292$, $p < .001$), and diabetes education ($r = .679$, $p < .001$) but not the other demographic variables medication type, level of education, marital status, and employment status, where $p > .05$.

Table 12. Correlations of Self-care management and Demographic variables

	Correlations								
	Variables	1	2	3	4	5	6	7	8
1	Combined Self-care Management	1.00	-0.08	.146*	.292**	0.04	-0.14	.679**	0.08
		-----	0.26	0.04	0.00	0.52	0.13	0.00	0.26
2	medication_type	-0.08	1.00	-.446	-.244	0.02	-0.11	-.182	0.02
		-----	0.00	0.01	0.85	0.21	0.04	0.83	0.83
3	duration_of_illness	-.446	1.00	.392	0.06	0.02	.260	0.10	0.10
		0.04	0.00	-----	0.00	0.44	0.86	0.00	0.21
4	age_group	.292	-.244	.392	1.00	0.11	0.07	.350	0.02
		0.00	0.01	0.00	-----	0.18	0.47	0.00	0.80
5	level_of_education	0.04	0.02	0.06	0.11	1.00	.201	0.10	0.00
		0.52	0.85	0.44	0.18	-----	0.02	0.26	0.96
6	marital_status	-0.11	-0.11	0.02	0.07	.201	1.00	-0.15	0.00
		0.13	0.21	0.86	0.47	0.02	-----	0.11	0.98
7	diabetes_education	.679	-.182	.260	.350	0.10	-0.15	1.00	0.11
		0.00	0.04	0.00	0.00	0.26	0.11	-----	0.22
8	employment_status	0.08	0.02	0.10	0.02	0.00	0.00	0.11	1.00
		0.26	0.83	0.21	0.80	0.96	0.98	0.22	-----

*. Correlation is significant at the 0.05 level (2-tailed)
**. Correlation is significant at the 0.01 level (2-tailed).

Table 13 illustrates a correlation of self-care knowledge and self-care management behaviors. Self-care knowledge and self-care management behaviors are an integral part of diabetes management. Self-care knowledge was moderately correlated but statistically significant with self-care management behaviors: Diet ($r = .178$, $p < .01$), Physical Activity ($r = .171$, $p < .05$), and Medications ($r = .149$, $p < .05$), but not Blood Glucose Testing ($r = .076$, $p = .270$) and Foot Care ($r = .105$, $p = .117$). A study conducted by Kugbe, Asante, and Adulai (2017) found a statistically significant positive correlation between diabetes knowledge and blood sugar testing ($r = .43$, $p < .001$) and foot care ($r = .18$, $p < .05$).

Table 13. Correlations of Self-care knowledge and Self-care management behaviors

	Self-care Management Behaviors				
	Diet	Physical Activity	Glucose Testing	Foot Care	Medications
Self-care knowledge score (Diabetes Knowledge)	178**	.171*	.076	.105	.149*
Kendall's tau b Coefficient Sig. (2-tailed)	.008	.013	.270	.117	.036
** $p < .01$, * $p < .05$					

Figure 6 is a histogram of self-care management scores. As shown in the figure, 60.83% of the scores are above the mean (78.58±17.986) and are skewed to the right, indicating a high degree of knowledge of self-care management among the sample.

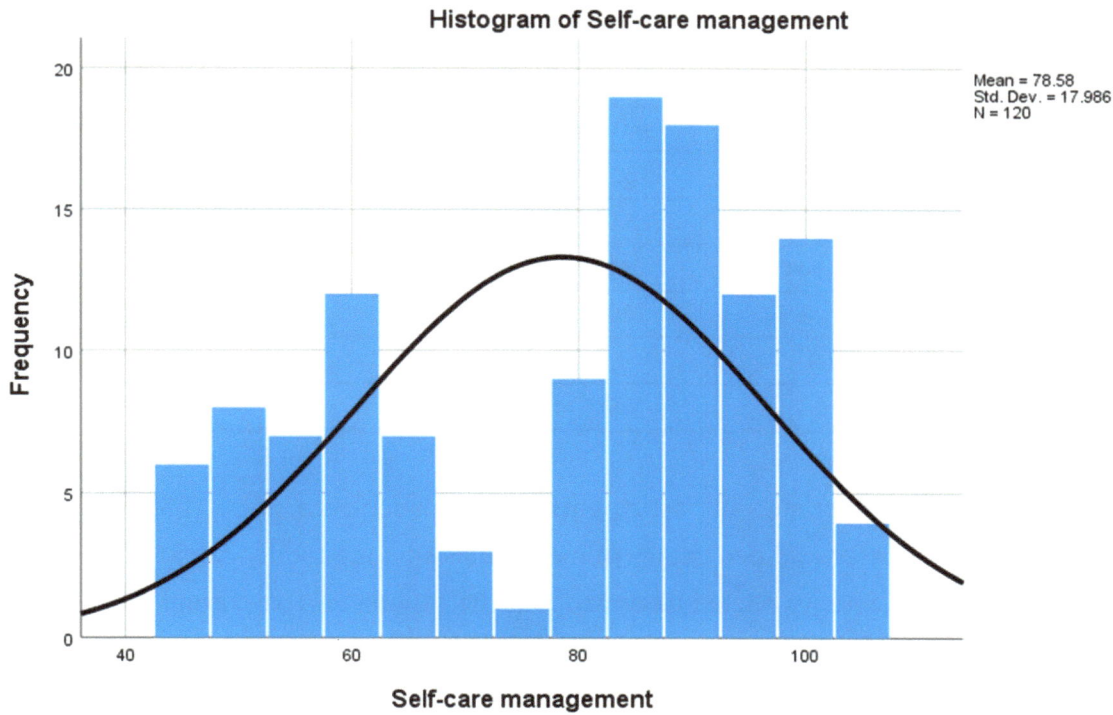

Figure 6. Histogram of Self-care management scores

Self-care Efficacy

Self-care efficacy was measured by an 8-item, 10-point Diabetes Self-care efficacy scale used in this study to assess how confident an individual is in performing activities related to their diabetes. Each answer scored 10 points for a total of 80 points. Self-efficacy was characterized into three categories: diet, exercise, and control self-efficacy. Control self-efficacy is the individual's confidence to engage in activities to control their diabetes, such as visiting the doctor when he or she feels threatened by symptoms of the disease. Table 14 is a descriptive statistics of self-care efficacy by categories. As shown in Table 13, more participants were confident in following their diet plan (16.50±7.899) than their exercise efficacy (15.71±4.661) and control efficacy (10.55±4.099).

Table 14. Descriptive Statistics of Self-care Efficacy

Self-care Efficacy Statistics				
		Diet	Exercise	Control	Combined Efficacy Store
N	Valid	120	120	120	120
	% Score	0	0	0	0
Mean		16.50	15.71	10.55	42.76
Median		16.00	16.00	11.00	43.00
Std. Deviation		4.964	4.661	4.099	7.899
Range		24	20	18	34
Minimum		4	5	2	25
Maximum		28	25	20	59

Table 15 illustrates the characteristics of participants with high self-care efficacy. Shown in each category in the table, is the number and percentage of individuals who are totally confident that he or she could complete the task or activity related to controlling their diabetes. For example, when asked "How confident do you feel that you can eat your meals every 4 to 5 hours every day, including breakfast every day?", 12 (10%) of individuals scored a maximum of 10 points, indicating their confidence in completing the task.

Table 15. Characteristics of Participants with High Self-care Efficacy Score

	Question	n	%[1]
1	How confident do you feel that you can eat your meals every 4 to 5 hours every day, including breakfast every day?	12	10.0
2	How confident do you feel that you can follow your diet when you have to prepare or share food with other people who do not have diabetes?	8	6.7
3	How confident do you feel that you can choose the appropriate foods to eat when you are hungry (for example, snacks)?	14	11.7
4	How confident do you feel that you can exercise 15 to 30 minutes, 4 to 5 times a week?	6	5.0
5	How confident do you feel that you can do something to prevent your blood sugar level from dropping when you exercise	14	11.7
6	How confident do you feel that you know what to do when your blood sugar level goes higher or lower than it should be?	10	8.3
7	How confident do you feel that you can judge when the changes in your illness mean you should visit the doctor?	11	9.2
8	How confident do you feel that you can control your diabetes so that it does not interfere with the things you want to do?	8	6.7

Table 16 illustrates the correlation table between self-care efficacy and the demographic variables. As shown, there is a moderate to strong correlation between self-care efficacy and level of education ($r = 0.185$, $p < .01$), and diabetes education ($r = 0.164$, $p < .05$), but not the other demographic variables where $p > .05$.

Table 16. Correlations of Self-care efficacy and Demographic variables

	Correlations								
	Variables	1	2	3	4	5	6	7	8
1	Combined Self-care Efficacy	1.00	-.0.08	0.12	0.14	.185**	.08	.164*	
		-----	0.27	0.08	0.08	0.01	0.32	0.03	0.94
2	medication_type	-0.08	1.00	-0.45	-0.24	0.02	-0.11	-0.18	0.02
		0.27	-----	0.00	0.01	0.85	0.21	0.04	0.83

** Correlation is significant at the .001 level (2-tailed)

* Correlation is significant at the .05 level (2-tailed).

	Correlations							
3	duration_of_illness	0.12	-0.44	1.00	0.39	0.06	0.02	0.26	0.10
		0.08	0.00	-----	0.00	0.44	0.86	0.00	0.21
4	age_group	0.14	-0.24	0.39	1.00	0.11	0.07	0.35	0.02
		0.08	0.01	0.00	-----	0.18	0.47	0.00	0.80
5	level_of_education	0.18	0.02	0.06	0.11	1.00	0.20	0.10	0.00
		0.01	0.85	0.44	0.18	-----	0.02	0.26	0.96
6	marital_status	0.08	-0.11	0.02	0.07	0.20	1.00	-0.15	0.00
		0.32	0.21	0.86	0.47	0.02	-----	0.11	0.98
7	diabetes_education	.164	-0.18	0.26	0.35	0.10	-0.15	1.00	0.11
		0.03	0.04	0.00	0.00	0.26	0.11	-----	0.22
8	employment_status	-0.01	0.02	0.10	0.02	0.00	0.00	0.11	1.00
		0.94	0.83	0.21	0.80	0.96	0.98	0.22	-----

** Correlation is significant at the .001 level (2-tailed)

* Correlation is significant at the .05 level (2-tailed).

Figure 7. is the histogram of the distribution of self-care efficacy scores.

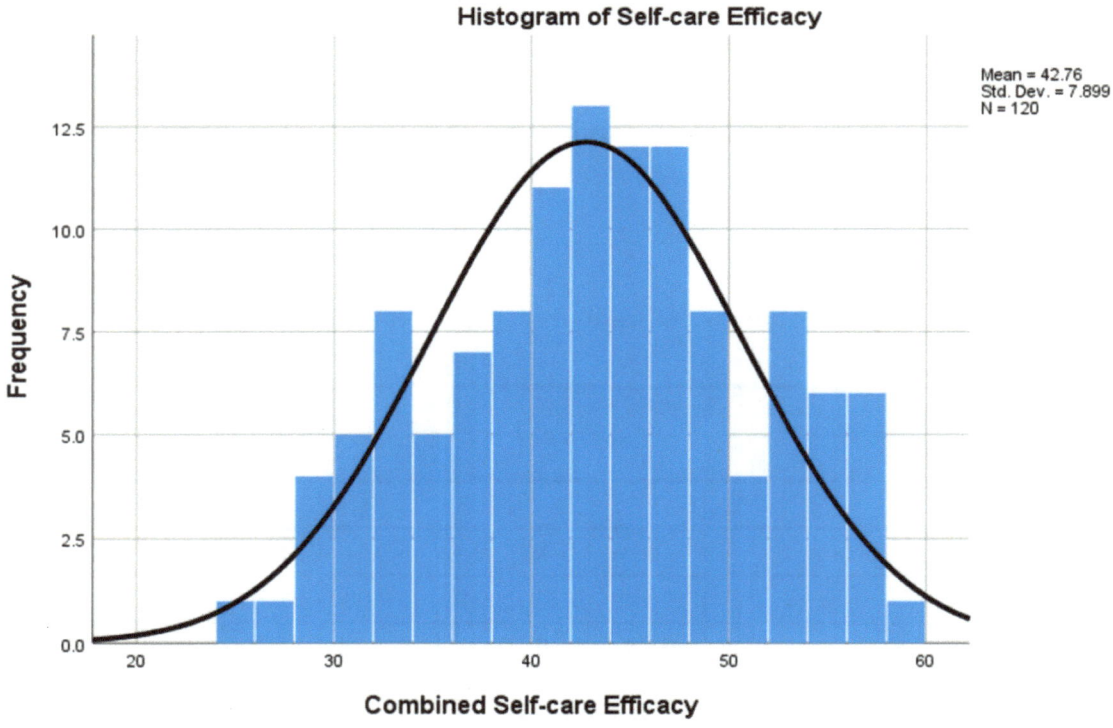

Figure 7. Distribution of the Self-care Efficacy Scale

Data Analysis

Data was collected from SurveyMonkey and downloaded into Microsoft Excel to check for outliers and missing data. A total of 120 participants selfidentified as middle-aged Black/African American women (45 to 64 years of age) with type 2 diabetes, and living in Dallas or Tarrant County, Texas, granted their assent for this study. The data were uploaded into SPSS version 25 for analysis. The data were analyzed using bi-variate correlation, Pearson chi-square test, Mann Whitney u-test, and binary logistic regression. Pearson's chi-square tests were performed to determine the significance of the categorical variables with $\alpha = .05$.

The first research question (RQ#1) was "What is the relationship, if any, between self-care efficacy and self-care knowledge in middle-aged Black/African-American women with T2DM, in north Texas?" The null hypothesis contends there was no significant relationship between self-care efficacy and self-care knowledge in middle-aged Black/African-American women with T2DM in north Texas. To address this hypothesis, a bivariate analysis was conducted to assess the association between the two variables. The results show a significant but low to moderate correlation between self-care efficacy and selfcare knowledge ($r = .172$, $p < 0.05$). Indicating that even though an increase in self-efficacy can positively increase self-care knowledge, the variables are not statistically related, $X^2(450, 120) = 474.037$, $p = 0.209$. Based on the evidence, the null hypothesis was rejected to state that there was a statistically significant relationship between self-care efficacy and self-care knowledge.

The second research question RQ#2) was "What is the relationship, if any, between self-care efficacy and self-care management in middle-aged Black/African-American women with T2DM, in north Texas?" The null hypothesis contends there is no significant relationship between self-care efficacy and self-care management in middle-aged Black/African-American women with T2DM, in north Texas." To address this hypothesis, a bivariate analysis was conducted to assess the significance of the association between the two variables. There was a statistically significant, but moderate correlation between self-care efficacy and self-care management ($r = .370$, $p < 0.001$). The results of a chisquare test of independence did not show a statistically strong evidence of a relationship, $X^2(1305, 120) = 1359.482$, $p = 0.143$. Based on the evidence, the null hypothesis was rejected to state that there was a statistically significant relationship between self-care efficacy and self-care management.

The third research question (RQ#3) was "What is the relationship, if any, between self-care knowledge and self-care management in middle-aged Black/African-American women with T2DM in north Texas?" The null hypothesis contends there is no significant relationship between self-care knowledge and self-care management in middle-aged Black/African-American women with T2DM, in north Texas." To address this hypothesis, a bivariate analysis was conducted to assess the significance of the association between the two variables. There was a moderate correlation between self-care knowledge and self-care management ($r = .172$, $p < .05$) indicating that people with self-care knowledge of diabetes were more likely to engage in self-care management even though there was no evidence of a statistically significant relationship, X^2 (450, 120) = 474.037, p = 0.209. Based on the evidence, the null hypothesis was rejected to state that there was a statistically significant relationship between selfcare knowledge and self-care management.

Lastly, a logistic regression was run to determine whether diabetes education (criterion variable) could be predicted by self-care knowledge, self-care management, self-care efficacy, and the demographic variables: medication type, duration of illness, age group, and level of education (predictor variables). All variables with a high P-level ($p > 0.10$) that were not statistically correlated with self-care knowledge were discarded and not entered into the model. Two variables that met such criteria were marital status (p = 0.231) and employment status (p = 0.887). Table 4.12 in Appendix J illustrates the contribution of each predictor variable to the model and its statistical significance.

Based on the Hosmer and Lemeshow Test for goodness of fit, the logistic regression model was a good fit, X^2 (8) = 2.92, $p < 0.935$ even though it is not statistically significant. Overall, the logistic regression model was statistically significant, X^2 (7) = 136.971, $p < 0.0005$. The model explained 68.1% (Cox and Snell R^2) to 91.2% (Nagelkerke R^2) variability in diabetes education, and correctly predicted 95.8% of all cases. Indicating that respondents who were engaged in self-care management were 2.951 times more likely to have had diabetes education training than those who did not. Self-care knowledge and self-care efficacy did not predict diabetes education. The demographic variables: mediation type, duration of illness, age group, and level of education did not statistically contribute to the model. Although not statistically significant, respondents with a longer duration of illness were 6.043 times more likely to have received diabetes education training. Respondents with higher education levels were 1.375 times more likely to have received diabetes education training. Likewise, a one unit increase in age was associated with a reduction in the likelihood of engaging in effective self-care management, and a one unit increase in medication type was associated with a reduction in the likelihood of engaging in effective self-care maintenance (Laerd Statistics, 2018).

Summary

Chapter 4 presented a summary of the data collected from SurveyMonkey and analyzed for 120 respondents using bivariate statistical analysis. Advertising flyers were posted at churches and public libraries. Upon meeting the inclusion criteria and signing the informed consent, prospective participants were given access to the survey. Prospective participants used their smart phones or a computer to access the survey on SurveyMonkey. Data were downloaded into Microsoft Excel and sanitized before uploading to the IBM SPSS software. Data were checked for linearity, multicollinearity, homoscedasticity, and for univariate outliers and normality. There were no significant multicollinearity found among the variables. A histogram was generated for all variables to assess the data for normality. Self-care knowledge and self-care efficacy did not deviate substantially from normality. However, self-care management was substantially skewed to the right, indicating a high degree of knowledge of self-care management among the sample.

The bivariate correlation using Kendall's tau correlation coefficient showed a statistically significant but low to moderate correlation between selfcare efficacy and self-care knowledge, a statistically significant but moderate correlation was shown between self-care efficacy and self-care management, and between self-care knowledge and self-care management. A Pearson chi-square test of independence, however, did not show a statistically strong evidence of a relationship between self-care knowledge and self-care efficacy, self-care knowledge and self-care management, and self-care efficacy and self-care management.

There was a moderate to strong correlation between self-care knowledge and the demographic variables: medication type, diabetes education, duration of illness, age, and education, but not marital status, and employment status. There was a moderate to strong correlation between self-care management and duration of illness, age, and diabetes education; but not medication type, education, marital status, and employment status. There was a moderate to strong correlations between self-care efficacy and education, and diabetes education; but not medication type, duration of illness, age, marital status, and employment status. A binary logistic regression model found self-care maintenance significantly predicted diabetes education. Chapter 5 contains the conclusion and recommendations and discusses the significant aspects of the study results.

CHAPTER 5

Conclusion and Recommendations

The purpose of this descriptive, quantitative, correlational study was to assess the association and magnitude of the relationship, if any, between diabetesrelated knowledge, self-care efficacy, and self-care management in middle-aged Black/African-American women (45 – 64 years of age) with T2DM in north Texas. Chapter 4 provided a quantitative descriptive correlation and the results of the study. The present chapter discusses the significance of the results and presents the findings and interpretations, the implications for the study, and makes recommendations for future research study.

Summary of the Findings

One hundred and twenty (120) participants were selected to participate in the online survey, which was hosted by SurveyMonkey. Three research questions were asked to determine the relationships of the variables self-care knowledge, self-care management, and self-care efficacy among middle-aged Black/African American women with T2DM, living in Dallas or Tarrant County, north Texas. The results showed that the scores on the self-care knowledge, self-care management, and self-care efficacy tests were above average compared with other studies in the literature (Table 4.2). The reason may have been attributed to the high number of college educated participants and the number of respondents who had received diabetes education classes. It is worth noting, however, that this is a cross-sectional data derived from middle-aged Black/African American women with T2DM, residing in north Texas. Therefore, the results of this study cannot be generalized to the middle-aged Black/African American women population.

Black/African Americans are a vulnerable population to chronic health issues such as diabetes, in part because of their biological risk factors and in-part due to their socioeconomic status (National Institutes of Health [NIH], 2018). Research has shown that Black/African Americans suffer a higher incidence of diabetes-related complications (Spanakis & Golden, 2014). Other research has attributed this high incidence and the prevalence of diabetes-related complications to low socioeconomic status for Black/African American women (Kaiser Family Foundation [KFF], 2016).

Four confounding variables that are commonly measured in relation to the prevalence, knowledge, and self-care of diabetes among Black/African American women with diabetes are age, educational level, house-hold income (SES), and body mass index (BMI, Signorello et al., 2007). The current study did not measure SES and BMI as confounding variables since SES is difficult to quantify and could be a proxy for a myriad of potential confounders, and BMI could not be obtained since this study was an online survey. Unarguably, however, there is a plethora of literature covering the effects of low SES and BMI on Black/African Americans with diabetes as a significant factor for health disparities. The current study, however, found education to be significantly associated with higher knowledge of diabetes self-care knowledge, self-care management, and self-care efficacy. These results are contrary to all published epidemiological studies found in the literature. A possible explanation is that the study population may have received or attended diabetes education classes or have higher levels of college education to fully understand the consequences of non-compliance with self-care management. Based on the results of the Kendall's tau correlation, a prediction model was built to assess whether self-care knowledge, self-care efficacy, and the demographic variables: medication type, duration of illness, age, and level of education were predictive of diabetes education. Marital status and employment status were discarded and not entered into the regression model because of their statistical significance to self-care knowledge ($p > .10$). Diabetes education was dichotomized into two categories ("Y" = received diabetes education, "N" = did not receive diabetes education). The model predicted respondents who engaged in effective self-care management were 2.951 times more likely to have received diabetes education training. Although age and education contributed significantly to the model, however, they were not statistically significant.

Borhaninejad et al. (2017) found in a cross-sectional study of elderly diabetic patients that education, income, and diabetic knowledge were significantly associated with higher self-care behaviors ($p < 0.001$). The researchers also found in a multiple regression model that diabetes knowledge could predict 57% of the variability in self-care behaviors. The findings are consistent with the current study indicating that the relationship between self-care knowledge and self-care management are statistically significant.

Findings and Interpretation

The following research questions were addressed:

RQ#1 -What is the relationship, if any, between self-care efficacy and selfcare knowledge in middle-aged Black/African-American women with T2DM in north Texas?

Findings and Interpretation: a bivariate correlation using Kendall's tau correlation coefficient showed a statistically significant but low to moderate correlation between self-care efficacy and self-care knowledge. However, a Pearson chi-square test of independence found no evidence of a statistically significant relationship. There is sufficient evidence in the literature supporting the association between self-care efficacy and self-care knowledge (Mehta et al. 2015), indicating that an increase in self-efficacy may translate to an increase in self-care knowledge and vice versa. Therefore, the findings in this study are consistent with studies in the literature.

RQ#2 - What is the relationship, if any, between self-care efficacy and self-care management in middle-aged Black/African-American women with T2DM in north Texas?

Findings and Interpretation: a bivariate correlation using Kendall's tau correlation coefficient showed a statistically significant but low to moderate correlation between self-care efficacy and self-care management. However, a Pearson chi-square test of independence found no evidence of a statistically significant relationship between the variables. There is sufficient evidence in the literature to support the assertion that higher self-efficacy may translate to higher self-care management skills (Merandy, Morgan, Lee, and Scherr (2017). Diabetes is a complex disease requiring social and family support for self-care maintenance. In some instances, patients may require shorter hospital stays implying that patients and family members may have less time to prepare and comprehend the information required of them for on-going self-care maintenance. Self-efficacy represents "beliefs in one's capabilities to organize and execute the course of action required to produce given attainments" (Bandura, 1997, p. 3). Improved self-efficacy can lead to successful changes in behavior, resulting in improved self-care skills (Bandura, 1977).

RQ#3 – What is the relationship between self-care knowledge and selfcare management in middle-aged Black/African-American women with T2DM in north Texas?

Findings and Interpretation: a bivariate correlation using Kendall's tau correlation coefficient showed a statistically significant but low to moderate correlation between self-care knowledge and self-care management. However, a Pearson chi-square test of independence found no evidence of a statistically significant relationship between the variables. The results are consistent with those found in Kugbe, Asante, and Adulai (2017), showing that a statistically significant relationship exists between diabetes knowledge and diabetes self-care practices ($r = .31$, $p < .001$). Another study by Dawson, Walker, and Egede (2017) found diabetes knowledge was significantly associated with self-care activities: general diet, 0.15 ($p = .004$) and foot care, -0.15 ($p = .004$). The results suggest that patients with higher diabetes self-care knowledge were more likely than those with lower self-care knowledge to engage in higher diabetes self-care management skills.

A bivariate correlation using Kendall's tau correlation coefficient showed a statistically significant but low to moderate correlation between self-care knowledge and the demographic variables: medication type, duration of illness, age, level of education, and diabetes education, but not marital status and employment status. The findings in this study are corroborated by Zowgar et al. (2018) who found diabetes knowledge was significantly associated with age ($p < 0.05$), level of education ($p < .001$), but not marital status ($p = 0.264$).

Strengths and Limitations

Several limitations were identified in this study. First, The study was limited to middle-aged Black/African women residing in Dallas or Tarrant County, north Texas. However, since the IP tracking system on SurveyMonkey was turned off to avoid collecting personal identifiable information from the participants, the geographic locations from where the participants accessed the survey on SurveyMonkey and the actual demographics of the participants could not be determined. Therefore, the threats of sampling bias, selection bias, testing bias, self-report bias, and internal validity may have affected this study.

Second, a limitation to this study include self-report by respondents. Several methods were used to recruit participants online; therefore, there are no assurances that the respondents had type II diabetes other than what was selfreported. Most respondents were approached at church settings and told about the diabetes study. Some were given a copy of the flyer while others received their information from the flyers posted on the church's bulletin boards. The only time the prospective participant was recruited to take the survey was if he or she met the inclusion criteria and consented to the study. Third, the research design limited the scope of the study. Except for the DKT and the demographic questionnaire, the self-efficacy scale and the SDSCA scale measured data on a Likert-type scale. Likert-type scales are close-ended and therefore, prevented the researcher from asking open-ended questions.

Fourth, the cross-sectional nature of the study may not be used to determine causality between the variables. Diabetes is a life-time progressive disease and therefore, requires on-going self-care maintenance. Since the study was limited to investigating the relationships between variables, no conclusions about how one variable influences the other was considered. Therefore, the crosssectional nature of the study cannot be used to analyze behavior over a period of time.

Fifth, the use of a convenience and snowball sampling methods may have diminished the generalizability of the outcome of the study to the entire Black/African American women population. Sixth, the lack of compensation may have caused response bias whereby the respondent may not have answered the questions accurately. Therefore, future researchers should carefully consider these limitations before drawing any conclusions about the outcome of the study.

Recommendations

Given the evidence found in this study, policy changes are recommended for the state of Texas to expand Medicaid health insurance coverage to all lowincome, uninsured, and underinsured Black/African American women in Texas to have access to quality health care under the ACA Medicaid expansion program. Studies show that over 5 million Texans are uninsured, and underinsured. Roughly 20% of eligible adults who are currently eligible for Medicaid are not covered by health insurance and Black/African Americans are disproportionately affected by inadequate quality healthcare due to the lack of affordable healthcare insurance (KFF, 2016).

The effect of inadequate health coverage or the limited access to affordable quality health care may contribute to long term psychosocial and behavioral dysfunctions on self-care behaviors among the at-risk individuals. Particularly among Black/African Americans who in spite of the pharmacologic interventions, have a 0.85% higher than average HbA1c scores, and lower selfcare efficacy compared to their non-Hispanic white counterparts (CDC, 2013, Spruill et al., 2013). Unequal access to healthcare pose not only a moral and ethical dilemma within the Black/African American communities, it contributes to poor quality of life of the individuals and of the communities, and further exacerbates increasing healthcare costs that could have profound implications for the overall quality of care experienced by all Texans.

For example, a news article released by the Center for Children and Families (CCF, 2018) reported that the rate of uninsured in Medicaid expansion states under the 2010 Affordable Care Act, fell to 16% in 2015 and 2016, down from 35% in 2008 through 2009. That is in contrast with the uninsured rate of 38% in non-Medicaid expansion states such as Texas. Another published article which study funded by the Robert Wood Johnson Foundation found the ACA in Medicaid expansion states dropped to 7% down from 15.3%, adding 9.7 million new participants through the Medicaid expansion program (American Journal of Managed Care [AJMC], 2018).

Therefore, extending Medicaid health insurance to low-income and underserved communities should be considered a healthcare priority because it could potentially reduce overall healthcare costs for states, improve productivity of the communities, reduce healthcare disparities, improve health literacy and mental illness, and reduce unnecessary emergency services and hospitalizations. For example, individuals with diabetes and healthcare coverage could engage in preventative care to reduce their risk of acquiring complications or pre-mature mortality. Individuals could also engage in healthcare learning to improve their knowledge of diabetes and other risk factors or to increase their self-efficacy for self-care management. While the results of this study were not robust, they are significant in identifying psychosocial characteristics predictive of engagement in self-care behaviors of middle-aged Black/African American women that may be used for further research.

Summary

Chapter 5 reviewed the results, presented a summary of the findings and made recommendations for future research. The specific aims of this study was to determine whether a statistically significant relationship exists between self-care knowledge and self-care efficacy, self-care knowledge and self-care management, and self-care management and self-care efficacy. The findings show a statistically significant relationship between the three variables. More importantly, the results indicate a high degree of self-care knowledge, self-care management, and selfcare efficacy skills among the respondents. Although the results are encouraging, however, it is not consistent with the literature because Black/African Americans are found to have lower self-care knowledge, lower self-care skills, and lower efficacy. The positive results may also have been influenced by a high degree of college educated respondents who may have received diabetes education classes. More research is needed before developing a culturally-based diabetes-related education program to target middle-aged Black/African Americans with diabetes irrespective of their demographic status.

Conclusions

Diabetes is a chronic illness, if left untreated, could potentially create adverse health-related complications for the individual including blindness, cardiovascular diseases, nephrology, peripheral neuropathy leading to lower extremity amputations, and premature mortality. Black/African Americans are more likely to develop complications from diabetes particularly due to the lack of knowledge, and low socioeconomic conditions which have been directly linked to lower self-care efficacy and poor self-care management skills.

The findings from this study indicate that middle-aged Black/African American women residing in north Texas with type II diabetes, have higher diabetes-related knowledge, self-care skills, and self-care efficacy. Although generally, these findings are not consistent with the literature. However, these positive findings could be attributed to variables `that are correlated with self-care knowledge such as age, level of education, diabetes education, duration of illness, and type of medications used to treat their illness. In the review of the literature, higher self-care knowledge was found to be positively correlated with key demographic variables such as age, diabetes education, duration of illness, and education. Those findings are consistent with the current study. For this reason, culturally-targeted diabetes-related education programs should be developed and aimed at all Black/African Americans who develop type II diabetes, irrespective of age and gender. Identifying Black/African-American women with adverse psychosocial deficits towards self-care behaviors in the early stages of diagnosis may have practical implications in the way culturally-flexible interventions are created to target the underlying causes and prevent further complications. The implication for this study may ascertain perceptions about barriers to self-care behaviors and may influence patient adherence and self-care efficacy for self-care behaviors, ultimately leading to better quality of life among this population.

REFERENCES

ADA (American Diabetes Association). (2012). Standards of medical care in diabetes - 2012. Retrieved from http://www.diabetes.org/

ADA (American Diabetes Association). (2013). Economic costs of diabetes in the U.S. in 2012. Retrieved from http://www.care.diabetesjournals.org/

AHA (American Heart Association). (2015). Sex differences in T2DM affect cardiovascular disease risk. Retrieved from http://newsroom.heart.org/news/sex-differences-in-type-2-diabetes-affectcardiovascular-disease-risk

Ahola, A. J., & Groop, P-H. (2012). Barrier to Self-care management of diabetes. *DIABETIC Medicine, 30*(4), 413-420. doi:10.1111/dme.12105

AJMC (American Journal of Managed Care). (2018). ACA pushed uninsured rate down to 10% in 2016, even more so in Medicaid expansion states. *American Journal of Managed Care.* Retrieved from https://www.ajmc.com/newsroom/aca-pushed-uninsured-rate-down-to-10in-2016-even-more-so-in-medicaid-expansion-states

Al Sayah, F., Majumdar, S. R., Egede, L. E., & Johnson, J. A. (2104). Measurement properties and comparative performance of health literacy screening questions in a predominantly low income African-American population with diabetes. *Patient Education and Counseling, 97*(1), 88-95. doi:10.1016/j.pec.2014.07.008

Al-Qazaz, H. Kh., Sulaiman, S. A., Hassali, M. A., Shafie, A. A., Sundram, S., Al-Nuri, R., & Saleem, F. (2011). Diabetes knowledge, medication adherence and glycemic control among patients with type 2 diabetes. *International Journal of Clinical Pharmacy, 33*(6), 1028-1034. doi:10.1007/s11096-011-9582-2

Auslander, W. F., Thompson, S., Dreitzer, D., White, N. H., & Santiago, J. V. (1997). Disparity in glycemic control and adherence between African American African-American and Caucasian youths with diabetes. *Diabetes Care, 20*(10), 1569-1575.

Barrera, M., & Garrison-Jones, C. V. (1988). Properties of the beck depression inventory as a screening instrument for adolescent depression. *Journal of Abnormal Child Psychology, 16*(3), 263-273. doi:10.1007/bf00913799.

Becker, M. H. (1974). The Health Belief Model and Personal Health Behavior. Health Education Monographs. Vol. 2 No. 4.

Becker, M. H., Radius, S. M., & Rosenstock, I. M. (1978). Compliance with a medical regimen for asthma: A test of the health belief model, *Public Health Reports, 93*, 268-77.

Bellis-Berry, J., Watson, C., Kadimpati, S., Crockett, S., Mohamed, E. A., & Davis, O. I. (2015). Black Men's perceptions and knowledge of diabetes:

A Church-affiliated barbershop focus group study. *Journal of Racial Ethnic Health Disparities, 2*(4), 465-472. doi:10.1007/s40615-015-0094-y Berkowitz, S. A., Meigs, J. B., & Wexler, D. J. (2013). Age at type 2 diabetes onset and glycaemic control: Results from the national health and nutrition examination survey (NHANES) 2005-2010. *Diabetologia, 56*(12), 2593-600. doi:http://dx.doi. org/10.1007/s00125-013-3036-4

Bhattacharya, G. (2012). Psychosocial impacts of type 2 diabetes self-care management in a rural African-American population. *Journal of Immigrant and Minority Health, 14*(6), 1071-1081. doi:10.1007/ s10903-012-9585-7

Bielamowicz, M. K., Pope, P., & Rice, C. A. (2013). Sustaining a creative community-based diabetes education program: Motivating Texans with type 2 diabetes to do well with diabetes control. *The Diabetes Educator, 39*(1), 119-127.

Billimek, J., Malik, S., Sorkin, D. H., Schmalbach, P., Ngo-Metzger, Q., Greenfield, S., & Kaplan, S. H. (2015). Understanding Disparities in Lipid Management Among Patients with Type 2 Diabetes: Gender Differences in Medication Nonadherence after Treatment Intensification. *Women's Health Issues, 25*(1), 6-12. doi.org/10.1016/j.whi.2014.09.004

Blascovich, J., Tomaka, J., Brennan, K., Kelsey, R. M., Hughes, P., Coad, M., & Adlin, R. (1992). Affect intensity and cardiac arousal. *Journal of Personality & Social Psychology, 63*(1), 164-174.

Bogner, H. R., Morales, K. H., Vries, H. F., & Cappola, A. R. (2012). Integrated management of type 2 diabetes mellitus and depression treatment to improve medication adherence: A randomized controlled trial. *Annals of Family Medicine, 10*(1), 15-22.

Borg, W. R., & Gall, M. D. (1996). *Educational research: An introduction* (6th ed.). New York, NY: Longman.

Bosch, M. L. V., Robbins, L. B., & Anderson, K. (2015). Correlation of physical activity in middle-aged women with and without diabetes. *Western Journal of Nursing Research, 37*(12), 1581-1603. doi:10.1177/0193945914541333

Bosomworth, N. J. (2013). Approach to identifying and managing atherogenic dyslipidemia. *Canadian Family Physician, 59*(11), 1169-1180.

Bowen, P. G., Clay, O. J., Lee, L. T., Vice, J., Ovalle, F., & Crowe, M. (2015). Association of social support and self-care efficacy with quality of life in older adults with diabetes. *Journal of Gerontological Nursing, 41*(12), 1-9.

Cavusoglu, H. (2001). Self-esteem in adolescence: A comparison of adolescents with diabetes mellitus and leukemia. *Pediatric Nursing, 27*(4), 355.

CCF (Center for Children and Families). (2018). Uninsured rates drop sharply in Medicaid expansion states. *Georgetown University Health Policy Institute.* Retrieved from https://ccf.georgetown. edu/2018/09/26/uninsured-ratesdropped-sharply-in-medicaid-expansion-states/

CDC (Center for Disease Control and Prevention). (2014a). Age-Adjusted Percentage of Adults with Diabetes Using Any Diabetes Medication, by Race/Ethnicity, United States, 1997–2011. Retrieved from http://www.cdc.gov/diabetes/statistics/meduse/fig5.htm

CDC (Center for Disease Control and Prevention). (2014b). Diabetes Report Card 2014. Atlanta, GA: Center for Disease Control and Prevention, U.S Department of Health and Human Services; 2015.

CDC (Center for Disease Control and Prevention). (2015). Summary Health Statistics. *National Health Interview Survey, 1997–2015*, Sample Adult Core component. Retrieved from https://www.cdc. gov/nchs/data/nhis/earlyrelease/earlyrelease201605_14.p df

CDC (Center for Disease Control and Prevention). (2015a). National Diabetes Fact Sheet, 2011. Retrieved from https://www.cdc.gov/diabetes/pubs/pdf/ndfs_2011.pdf

Chao, J., Nau, D. P., Aikens, J. E., & Taylor, S. D. (2005). The mediating role of health beliefs in the relationship between depressive symptoms and medication adherence in persons with diabetes. *Research in Social and Administrative Pharmacy, 1*, 508-525. doi:10.1016/j.sapharm.2005.09.002

Charteris-Black, J. (2012). Shattering the Bell Jar: Metaphor, Gender, and Depression. *Metaphor & Symbol, 27*(3), 199-216.

Chen, A. M. H., Yehle, K. S., Albert, N. M., Ferraro, K. F., Mason, H. L., Murawski, M. M., & Plake, K. S. (2014). Relationships between health literacy and heart failure knowledge, self-care efficacy, and self-care adherence. *Research in Social & Administrative Pharmacy : RSAP, 10*(2), 378–386. http://doi.org/10.1016/j.sapharm.2013.07.001

Chen, G., Qin, L., & Ye, J. (2014). Leptin levels and risk of type 2 diabetes: gender-specific meta-analysis. *Obesity Reviews, 15*(2), 134-142. doi:10.1111/obr.12088

Chew, B.-H., Shariff-Ghazali, S., & Fernandez, A. (2014). Psychological aspects of diabetes care: Effecting behavioral change in patients. *World Journal of Diabetes, 5*(6), 796–808. http://doi.org/10.4239/wjd.v5.i6.796

Chlebowy, D. O., Hood, S., & LaJoie, A. S. (2013). Gender differences in diabetic self-care management among African American African-American adults. *Western Journal of Nursing Research, 35*(6), 703-721.

Choudhury, S., Hussain, S., Yao, G., Hill, J., Malik, W., & Taheri, S. (2013). The impact of a diabetes local enhanced service on quality outcome framework diabetes outcomes. *PLOS ONE, 8*(12), 1-7.

Christie-Mizell, C. A., Blount, S. A., Pirtle, W. N. L., Dagadu, H. E., Leslie, E. T. A., & Vielehr, M. A. (2015). Psychiatric medication, African-Americans and the paradox of mistrust. *Journal of the National Medical Association, 107*(2), 51-59.

CHS (Center for Health Statistics). (2010). North Texas Behavioral Risk Factor Surveillance System Survey Data

CHS (Center for Health Statistics). (2012). Texas Behavioral Risk Factor Surveillance System Survey Data. Austin, Texas: *Texas Department of State Health Services*, 2011-2014. Retrieved from https://www.dshs.texas.gov/chs/brfss/query/brfss_form.shtm

Cohen, J. (1988). *Statistical Power Analysis for the Behavioral Sciences,* (2nd ed.). Hillsdale, NJ: Erlbaum.

Cosansu, G., & Erdogan, S. (2014). Influence of psychosocial factors on self-care behavior and glycemic control in Turkish patients with type 2 diabetes mellitus. *Journal of Transcultural Nursing, 25*(1), 51-59. doi:10.1177/1043659613504112

Dall, T. M., Zhang, Y., Chen, Y. J., Quick, W. W., Yang, W. G., & Fogli, J. (2010). The economic burden of diabetes. *Health Affairs, 29*(2), 297-303. doi:10.1377/hithaff.2009.0155 de Groot, M., Kushnick, M., Doyle, T., Merrill, J., McGlynn, M., Shubrook, J., & Schwartz, F. (2010). Depression among adults with diabetes: Prevalence, impact, and treatment options. *Diabetes Spectrum, 23*(1), 15-18.

Dismuke, C. E., & Egede, L. E. (2010). Association between major depression, depressive symptoms and personal income in US adults with diabetes. *General Hospital Psychiatry, 32*, 484-491. doi:10.1177/0145721705280414

Egede, L. E., Grubaugh, A. L., & Ellis, C. (2010). The effect of major depression on preventive care and quality of life among adults with diabetes. *General Hospital Psychiatry, 32*, 563-569.

Eisenstat, S. A., Ulman, K., Siegel, A. L., Carlson, K. (2013). Diabetes group visits: Integrated medical care and behavioral support to improve diabetes care and outcomes from a primary care perspective. *Current Diabetes Reports, 13*(2), 177-187. doi:10.1007/s11892-012-0349-5

Elliott, A. J., Harris, F., & Laird, S. G. (2016). Patients' beliefs on the impediments to good diabetes control: A mixed methods study of patients in general practice. *British Journal of General Practice*, 913-919. doi:10.3399/bjgp16X687589

Fox, C. S., Golden, S. H., Anderson, C., Bray, G. A., Burke, L. E., de Boer, H., & Vafiadis, D. K. (2015). Update on prevention of cardiovascular disease in adults with type 2 diabetes mellitus in light of recent evidence: A scientific statement from the American Heart Association and the American Diabetes Association. *Circulation*, Retrieved from https://doi.org/10.1161/CIR.0000000000000230

Funnell, M. M., Brown, T. L., Childs, B. P., Haas, L. B., Hosey, G. M., Jensen, B., & Weiss, M. A. (2010). National Standards for Diabetes SelfManagement Education. *Diabetes Care, 33*(Suppl 1), S89–S96. http://doi.org/10.2337/dc10-S089

Glanz, K., Marcus Lewis, F. & Rimer, B. K. (1997). Theory at a Glance: A Guide for Health Promotion Practice. National Institute of Health.

Glanz, K., Rimer, B. K. & Lewis, F. M. (2002). Health Behavior and Health Education. Theory, Research and Practice. San Fransisco: Wiley & Sons

Grochowska-Niedworok, E., Brukalo, K., Kardas, M., & Calyniuk, B. (2015). Contribution of environmental risk factors including lifestyle to inequalities non-communicable (Chronic) diseases such as diabetes. *European Journal of Sustainable Development, 4*(2), 113-120.

Guariguata, L., Whiting, D. R., Hambelton, I., Beagley, J., Linnenkamp, U., & Shaw, J. E. (2014). Global estimates of diabetes prevalence for 2013 and projections for 2035, *Diabetes Research and Clinical Practice, 103*(2), 137–149. doi:10.1016/j.diabres.2013.11.002

Gucciardi, E., Fortugno, M., Senchuk, A., Beanlands, H., McCay, E., & Peel, E. E. (2013). Self-monitoring of blood glucose in black Caribbean and South Asian Canadians with non-insulin treated type 2 diabetes mellitus: A qualitative study of patients' perspectives. *BioMed Central Endocrine Disorders, 13*(1), 1-10.

Hauke, J. & Kossowski, T. (2011). Comparison of values of Pearson's and Spearman's Correlation Coefficient on the same sets of data. *QUAESTIONES GEOGRAPHICAE 30*(2). Retrieved from http://geoinfo.amu.edu.pl/qg/archives/2011/QG302_087-093.pdf Hayes, W. L. (1973). *Statistics for the Social Sciences* (2nd ed.). New York: Holt, Rinehart and Winston.

IDF (International Diabetes Federation). (2012). The economic impact of diabetes. Retrieved from http://www.idf.org/diabetesatlas/economicimpacts-diabetes

Kirsh, S., Hein, M., Pogach, L., Schectman, G., Stevenson, L., Watts, S., Radhakrishnan, A., Chardos, J., & Aron, D. (2012). Improving outpatient diabetes care. *American Journal of Medical Quality, 27*(3), 233-240.

Kootte, R. S., Vrieze, A., Holleman, F., Dallinga-Thie, G. M., Zoetendai, E. G., de Vos, W. M., & Nieuwdorp, M. (2012). The therapeutic potential of manipulating gut microbiota in obesity and type 2 diabetes mellitus. *Diabetes, Obesity & Metabolism, 14*(2), 112-120. doi:10.1111/j.1463-1326.2011.01483.x

Korbel, L., & Spencer, J. D. (2015). Diabetes mellitus and infections: An evaluation of hospital utilization and management costs in the United States. *Journal of Diabetes and Its Complications, 29*(2), 192-195.

Kordas, K., Ardoino, G., Ciccariello, D., Manay, N., Ettimger, A. S., Cook, C. A., & Queirolo, E. L. (2011, Dec.). Association of maternal and child blood lead and hemoglobin levels with maternal perceptions of parenting their young children. *Neurotoxicology, 32*(6), 693-701.

Kowitt, S. D., Urlaub, D., Guzman-Corrales, L., Mayer, M., Ballesteros, J., Graffy, J., Simmons, D., Cummings, D. M., & Fisher, E. B. (2015). Emotional support for the diabetes management; An international crosscultural study. *The Diabetes EDUCATOR, 41*(3). 291-300. doi:10.1177/0145721715574729

Laranjo, L., Neves, A. L., Costa, A., Ribeiro, R. T., Couto, L., & Sa, A. B. (2015). Facilitators, barriers and expectations in the self-care management of type 2 diabetes - A qualitative study from Portugal. *European Journal of General Practice, 21*(2), 103-110.

Levin, L. S. (1983). Self-care in health. Department of Epidemiology and Public Health, School of Medicine, Yale University. Ann. Rev. Public Health. 4:181-201

Lustman, P. J., Gavard J. A. (2000). Psychosocial aspects of diabetes in adult populations. In: National Diabetes Data Group. *Diabetes in America* (2nd ed.). Bethesda (MD): National Institutes of Health, *National Institute of Diabetes and Digestive and Kidney Diseases*; 507-18

Masaku, K., Kalawale, B., & Mumec, J. (2008). Depression, anxiety and quality of life among diabetic patients: a comparative study. *Journal of National Medical Association, 100*, 73–8.

Mathew, R., Gucciardi, E., De Melo, M., & Barata, P. (2012). Self-care management experience among men and women with type 2 diabetes mellitus: A qualitative analysis. *BioMed Central Family Practice, 13*(1), 1-12.

Mayer-Davis, E. J., Beyer, J., Bell, R. A., Dabella, D., D'Agostino, R., Imperatore, G., Lawrence, J. M., & Rodriguez, B., 2009). Diabetes in African-American youth: Prevalence, incidence, and clinical characteristics: The search for diabetes in youth study. *Diabetes Care, 32*(Suppl. 2). 112-122. doi:10.2337/dc09-S203

McCambridge, J., Witton, J., & Elbourne, D. R. (2014). Systematic review of the Hawthorne effect: New concepts are needed to research participation effects. *Journal of Clinical Epidemiology, 67*(3), 267-277. doi:10.1016/j.jclinepi.2013.08.015

Merandy, K., Morgan, M. A., Lee, R., & Scherr, D. S. (2017). Improving selfefficacy and self-care in adult patients with urinary diversion: A pilot study. *Oncology Nursing Forum, 44*(3), E90-E100. doi:10.1188/17.ONF.E90-E100

Montague, M. C., Nichols, S. A., & Dutta, A. P. (2005, September/October) Selfcare management in African-American women with diabetes. *The Diabetes Educator, 31*(5).

Moreno-Indias, I., Cardona, F., Tinahones, F. J., & Queipo-Ortuno, M. I. (2014). Impact of the gut microbiota on the development of obesity and type 2 diabetes mellitus. *Frontiers in Microbiology, 5*, 1-10. doi:10.3389/fmicb.2014.00190

Mulder, B. C., van Belzen, M., Lokhorst, A. M., van Woerkum, C. M. J. (2015). Quality assessment of practice nurse communication with type 2 diabetes patients. *Patient Education and Counseling, 98*(2), 156-161.

NCHS (National Health Interview Survey). (2016). Summary Health Statistics: *National Health Interview Survey: 2014. Table A-4.* Retrieved from http://www.cdc.gov/nchs/nhis/shs/tables.htm

Nicklett, E. J., & Damiano, S. K. (2014). Too little, too late: Socioeconomic disparities in the experience of women living with diabetes. *Qualitative Social Work, 13*(3), 372-388. doi:10.1177/1473325014522572

Nicolucci, A., Burns, K. K., Holts, R. I. G., Comaschi, M., Hermanns,. N., Ishii, H., Kokoszka, A., Pouwer, F., Skovlund, S. E., Stuckey, H., Tarkun, I., Vallis, M., Wen, J., & Peyrot, M. (2013). Diabetes attitudes, wishes and needs second study (DAWN2): Cross-national benchmarking of diabetesrelated psychosocial outcomes for people with diabetes. *DIABETIC Medicine, 30*(7), 767-777.

NIH (National Institutes of Health). (2018). Factors contributing to higher incidence of diabetes for black Americans. Retrieved from https://www.nih.gov/news-events/nih-research-matters/factorscontributing-higher-incidence-diabetes-black-americans

OECD (Organization for Economic Cooperation and Development). (2017), "Diabetes care", in Health at a Glance 2017: OECD Indicators, *OECD Publishing, Paris.* doi:http://dx.doi.org/10.1787/health_glance-2017-32enhttp://dx.doi.org/10.1787/health_glance-2017-32-en

Oftedal, B., Bru, E., & Karlsen, B. (2011). Motivation for diet and exercise management among adults with type 2 diabetes. *Scandinavian Journal of Caring Science, 25*(4), 735-744. doi:10.1111/j.1471-6712.211.00884.x

Olson, E. A., & McAuley, E. (2015). Impact of a brief intervention on selfregulation, self-care efficacy and physical activity in older adults with type 2 diabetes. *Journal of Behavioral Medicine, 38*(6). 886-898. doi:10.1007/s10865-015-9660-3

Osborn, C. Y., Mayberry, L. S., Wagner, J. A., & Welch, G. W. (2014). Stressor may compromise medication adherence among adults with diabetes and low socioeconomic status. *Western Journal of Nursing Research, 36*(9), 1091-1110. doi:10.1177/0193945914524639

Polonsky, W. H. (2015). Poor medication adherence in diabetes: What's the problem? *Journal of Diabetes, 7*(6), 777-778. doi:10.1111/1753- 0407.12306

Poolsup, N., Suksomboon, N., & Kyaw, A. M. (2013). Systematic review and meta-analysis of the effectiveness of continuous glucose monitoring (CGM) on glucose control in diabetes. *Diabetology & Metabolic Syndrome, 5*, 1-14. doi:http://dx.doi.org/10.1186/1758-5996-5-39

Ricc-Cabello, I., Ruiz-Perez, I., Nevot-Cordero, A., Rodriguez-Barranco, M., Sordo, L., & Concalves, D. C. (2013). Health care interventions to improve the quality of diabetes care in African-Americans. *Diabetes Care, 36*(3), 760-768. doi:10.2337/dc12-1057

Rice, C. A. (2005, November – December). Prevention: The most economical way to manage diabetes. *Nursing Economics, 23*(6), 327.

Rosenstock, I. (1974). Historical Origins of the Health Belief Model. *Health Education Monographs.* Vol. 2 No. 4.

Rothman, R. L., Mulvaney, S., Elasy, T. A., VanderWoude, A., Gebretsadik, T., Shintani, A., Schlundt, D. (2008). Self-care management behaviors, racial disparities, and glycemic control among adolescents with type 2 diabetes. [Research Support, N.I.H., Extramural]. *Pediatrics, 121*(4), 912-919. doi:10.1542/peds.2007-1484

Runyon, M. K., Steer, R. A., & Deblinger, E. (2009). Psychometric characteristics of the Beck Self-Concept Inventory for youth with adolescents who have experienced sexual abuse. *Journal of Psychopathology & Behavioral Assessment, 31*(2), 129-136. doi:10.1007/s10862-008-9100-6

Ryan, J. G., Schwartz, R., Jennings, T., Fedders, M., & Vittoria, I. (2013). Feasibility of an internet-based intervention for improving diabetes outcome among low-income patients with a high risk for poor diabetes outcomes followed in a community clinic. *The Diabetes Educator, 39*(3), 365-375.

Salkind, Rosenthal, R. & Rubin, D. B. (1982). A simple, general-purpose display of magnitude of experimental effect. *Journal of Educational Psychology, 74*, 166-169.

Sapkota, S., Brie, J., Greenfield, J., & Aslani, P. (2015). A systematic review of interventions addressing adherence to anti-diabetic medications in patients with type 2 diabetes - impact on adherence. *PLoS ONE, 10*(2), 1-17. doi:10.1371/journal.pone.0118296

Sattar, N. (2013). Gender aspects in type 2 diabetes mellitus and cardiometabolic risk. *Best Practice & Research Clinical Endocrinology & Metabolism, 27*, 501–507.

Schneider, A. C., Lazo, M., Ndumele, C. E., Pankow, J. S., Coresh, J., Clark, J. M., & Selvin, E. (2013). Liver enzymes, race, gender and diabetes risk: The Atherosclerosis Risk in Communities (ARIC) Study. *Diabetic Medicine, 30*(8), 926-933. doi:10.1111/dme.12187

Schofied, D., Cunich, M. C., Shrestha, R. N., Passey, M. E., Veerman, L., Callander, E. J., Kelly, S. J., & Tanton, R. (2014). The economic impact of diabetes through; lost labour force participation on individual and government: Evidence from a microsimulation model. *BioMed Central Public Health, 14*(1), 1-8.

Sebastián Manzanares, G., Angel Santalla, H., Irene Vico, Z., López Criado, M. S., Alicia Pineda, L., & José Luis Gallo, V. (2012). Abnormal maternal body mass index and obstetric and neonatal outcome. *The Journal of Maternal-Fetal & Neonatal Medicine: The Official Journal of The European Association of Perinatal Medicine, The Federation of Asia And Oceania Perinatal Societies, The International Society of Perinatal Obstetricians, 25*(3), 308-312. doi:10.3109/1476 7058.2011.575905

Seo, D., Torabi, M. R., Li, K., John, P. M., Woodcox, S. G, & Perera, B. (2008). Perceived susceptibility to diabetes and attitudes towards preventing diabetes among college students at a large Midwestern University. *American Journal of Health Studies, 23*(3), 143-150.

Shakil, A., Church, R. J., & Rao, S. S. (2008). Gastrointestinal complications of diabetes. *American Family Physician, 77*(12), 1697-1702.

Shapiro, J. K. (2011). Correlation. Encyclopedia of Survey Research Methods. *Sage Publications, 155-156.* doi:http://dx.doi.org/10.4135/9781412963947

Sharma, A. M., & Lau, D. C. W. (2013). Obesity and type 2 diabetes mellitus. *Canadian Journal of Diabetes, 37*(2), 63-64.

Sharma, M., Nazareth, I., & Petersen, I. (2016). Trends in incidence, prevalence and prescribing in type 2 diabetes mellitus between 2000 and 2013 in primary care: A retrospective cohort study. *British Medical Journal, 6*(1), 1-8. doi:10.1136/bmjopen-2015- 010210

Shrivastava, S. R., Shrivastava, P. S., & Ramasamy, J. (2013). Role of self-care in management of diabetes mellitus, *Journal of Diabetes & Metabolic Disorders*, 12:14, https://jdmdonline.biomedcentral. com/articles/10.1186/2251-6581-12-14.

Signorello, L. B., Schlundt, D. G., Cohen, S. S., Steinwandel, M. D., Buchowski, M. S., McLaughlin, J. K., Hargreaves, M. K., & Blot, W. J. (2007). Comparing diabetes prevalence between African-Americans and whites of similar socioeconomic status. *American Journal of Public Health, 97*(12), 2260-2267.

Sims, M., Diez Roux, A. V., Boykin, S., Sarpong, D., Gebreab, S. Y., Wyatt, S. B., Hickson, D., Payton, M., Ekunwe, L., & Taylor, H. A. (2011). The socioeconomic gradient of diabetes prevalence, awareness, treatment, and control among African-Americans in the Jackson heart study. *Annals of Epidemiology, 21*(12), 892-898. doi:10.1016/j.annepidem.2011.05.006

Spanakis, E. K., & Golden, S. H. (2013). Race/ethic differences in diabetes and diabetic complications. *Current Diabetes Report, 13*, 814-823. doi:10.1007/s11892-013-0421-9

Spellman, C. W. (2009). Achieving glycemic control: Cornerstone in the treatment of patients with multiple metabolic risk factors. *The Journal of American osteopathic Association, 109*(Suppl. 1). Retrieved from http://www.jaoa.org/content/109/5_suppl_1/S8.full

Steer, R., Kumar, G., Beck, A., & Beck, J. (2005). Dimensionality of the Beck Youth Inventories with Child Psychiatric Outpatients. *Journal of Psychopathology & Behavioral Assessment, 27*(2), 123-131. doi:10.1007/s10862-005-5386-9

Steinbekk, A., Rygg, L. O., Lisulo, M., Rise, M. B., & Fretheim, A. (2012). Group based diabetes self-care management education compared to routine treatment for people with type 2 diabetes mellitus. A systematic review with meta-analysis. *BioMed Central Health Services Research, 12*(1), 1-19.

Stoop, C. H., Spek, V. RM., Pop, V. JM., Pouwer, F. (2011). Disease management for co-morbid depression and anxiety in diabetes mellitus: design of a randomised controlled trial in primary care. *BMC Family Practice, 12*(1), 139-144. doi:10.1186/1471-2296-12-139 van der Heijden, M., Pouwer, F., Romeijnders, A. C., & Pop, V. (2012). Testing the effectiveness of a self-care efficacy based exercise intervention for inactive people with type 2 diabetes mellitus: Design of a controlled clinical trial. *BioMed Central, 12*(1), 2-8.

Weymann, N., Dirmaier, J., von Wolff, A., Kriston, L., & Harter, M. (2015). Effectiveness of a web-based tailored interactive health communication application for patients with type 2 diabetes or chronic low back pain: Randomized controlled trial. *Journal of Medical Internet Research, 17*(3), 1-21.

Weymann, N., Harter, M., Petrak, F., Dirmaier, J. (2013). Health information, behavior change, and decision support for patients with type 2 diabetes: development of a tailored, preference-sensitive health communication application. *Patient Preference and Adherence, 7*, 1091-1099.

Whiting, D. R., Guariguata, L., Weil, C., Shaw, J. (2011). IDF diabetes atlas: Global estimates of the prevalence for 2011 and 2030. *Diabetes Research and Clinical Practice, 94*, 311-321. doi:10.1016/j.diabres.2011.10.029

WHO (World Health Organization). (2018). Gender and women's mental health. Gender disparities and mental health: The Facts. Retrieved from http://www.who.int/mental_health/prevention/genderwomen/en/

Wild, S., Roglic, G., Green, A., Sicree, R., & King, H. (2004). Global prevalence of diabetes: Estimates for the year 2000 and projections for 2030. *Diabetes Care, 27*(5), 1047-1053.

Wilkinson, A., Whitehead, L., & Ritchie, L. (2014). Factors influencing the ability to self-manage diabetes for adults living with Type I or 2 diabetes. *International Journal of Nursing Studies, 51*(1), 111-122. doi:http://dx.doi.org/10.1016/j.ijnurstu.2013.01.006

Williams, J. (2011). Good leadership can improve diabetes care for older people with diabetes. *Journal of Diabetes Nursing, 15*(2), 69.

Williams, S. A., Shi, L., Brenneman, S. K., Johnson, J. C., Wegner, & Fonseca, V. (2012). The burden of hypoglycemia on healthcare utilization, cost, and quality of life among type 2 diabetes mellitus patients. *Journal of Diabetes and Its Complications, 26*(5), 399-406. doi:10.1016/j.jdiacomp.2012.05.002

Windle, M., & Windle, R. C. (2013). Recurrent depression, cardiovascular disease, and diabetes among middle-aged and older adult women. *Journal of Affective Disorders, 150*, 895-902.

Xu, L., Jiang, C. Q., Schooling, C. M., Zhang, W. S., Cheng, K. K., & Lam, T. H. (2017). Liver enzymes as mediators of association between obesity and diabetes: The Guangzhou Biobank cohort study. *Annals of Epidemiology, 27*(3), 204-207.

Zhou, Q., Remsburg, R., Caufield, K., & Itote, E. W. (2012). Lifestyles behaviors, chronic diseases, and ratings of health between black and white adults with pre-diabetes. *The Diabetes EDUCATOR, 38*(2), 219-228. doi:10.1177/0145721712440334

Zoumenou, V. M., Himburg, S., Magnus, M., Johnson, L. S., & Adoueni, V. (2009). Measure of strength of commitment to successful diabetes selfcare management among blacks: Reliability and validity. *European Journal of Scientific Research, 26*(2), pp. 176-188. Retrieved from EBSCOhost.

Zowgar, A. M., Siddiqui, M. I., & Alattas, K. M. (2018). Level of diabetes knowledge among adult patients with diabetes using diabetes knowledge test. *Saudi Medical Journal, 39*(2).

Zulman, D. M., Rosland, A-M., Choi, H., Langa, K. M., & Heisler, M. (2012). The influence of diabetes psychosocial attributes and self-care management practices on change in diabetes status. *Patient Education and Counseling, 87*, 74-80. doi:10.1016/j.pec.2011.07.013

Appendix A

Advertising Flyer

I AM ASKING FOR YOUR HELP

Be a part of an important Diabetes Study for People with Type 2 Diabetes.

- ✓ Are you between 45 and 64 years of age?
- ✓ Have you been diagnosed with Type-II diabetes?
- ✓ Are you Black/African-American female?
- ✓ Do you live in Dallas County or Tarrant County, Texas?

If you answered **YES** to all these questions you may be eligible to participate in a diabetes research study of middle-aged Black/African-American women with **Type-II diabetes.** The study takes only 30 minutes to complete.

This is an investigational study to assess the knowledge of middle-aged Black/African American women with diabetes and to evaluate their ability to engage in effective self-care management of their disease. This study is completely voluntary. You may choose to withdraw from the study at any time without any risk to you. Your identity will not be made public. We do not ask for or collect any personal information from you. No medications will be given. This study will be available online 24/7 days a week for your convenience.

The study is being conducted in the state of Texas for residents of Dallas County or Tarrant County, Texas only. If you are willing to participate in this important research study, please go to https://www.surveymonkey.com/r/vicdenor.

Contact: Victor Akhidenor
Phone: **281-989-8293**
Email: vicdenor@gmail.com

APPENDIX B

Letter of Informed Consent

Dear Participant,

I am a student at the University of Phoenix working on a doctoral degree in Healthcare Administration. I am conducting a research study titled "Exploring Psychosocial Behaviors in Middle-aged Black/ African-American Women with Type-II Diabetes in North Texas.

The purpose of this study is to assess your capacity to effectively manage your diabetes.

To be eligible to participate in this study, you must be a Black/African-American female gender, have a medical diagnosis of Type-II diabetes mellitus, be between 45 – 64 years of age, and reside in north Texas (Dallas County or Tarrant County).

This study will NOT require you to be physically present to answer the survey questions. The survey questions will be provided on our electronic platform SurveyMonkey® to take at your convenience 24/7 days a week.

Your participation in this study is voluntary and appreciated. If you choose not to continue to participate, you may withdraw from the study at any time on the SurveyMonkey® platform. No penalty or risk of confidentially will be a result of any withdrawal. The results of the research study may be published **but** your name or identity will not appear in the published result. The researcher will use the information provided in a manner to avoid compromising or suggesting your identity. The researcher and his committee members and SurveyMonkey are the only ones to have access to the data. The data will be kept in a vault for three years after which it will be shredded.

I invite you to carefully read the <u>SurveyMonkey Privacy Policy</u>, which sets out in which context any personal data collected from you in the survey may be transferred to various countries, including the United States and other locations SurveyMonkey has offices.

In this research, there are no foreseeable risks to you. A possible benefit from this study is that it may help healthcare practitioners, policy makers, and others within the field of healthcare to craft policies to mitigate the effects of disparities in care for individuals affected by diabetes.

If you have questions at any time during the study please call me at 281-989-8293 or email to vicdenor@

email.phoenix.edu. You can also reach my dissertation Chair, Craig Follins, Ph.D., via email at cfollins@ email.phoenix.edu. For questions about your rights as a study participant, concerns or complaints please contact the University of Phoenix Institutional Review Board via email at researchhub@phoenix.edu.

It is important for you to know that:

1. Your participation is voluntary.

2. **You may decide to leave at any time.**

3. **I will keep your research records in locked cabinets and secure computer files.**

4. **The information you provide in this survey will be destroyed after three years.**

5. **The results may be published.**

By signing this form I acknowledge that I understand the nature of the study, the potential risks to me as a participant, and the means by which my identity will be kept confidential. My signature on this form also indicates that I am at least 18 years old and that I give my permission to voluntarily serve as a participant in the study described.

Victor Akhidenor - Researcher

Phone: 281-989-8293

I have read and agree to the above Consent Agreement   YES____   NO____

APPENDIX C

Demographic Questionnaire

Please provide all answers in this questionnaire to the best of your ability

1. **Are you Black/African American Female?**

   ☐ Yes ☐ No

2. **Do you use insulin and/or medication (pills)?**

   ☐ Insulin and Medications (pills)
   ☐ Insulin only
   ☐ Medications (pills) only
   ☐ None

3. **How long have you had Diabetes?**

   ☐ 1 to 4 Years ☐ 5 - 10 Years ☐ 11 - 15 Years ☐ Over 15 Years

4. **What is your age group?**

   ☐ Under 18 ☐ 18-24 ☐ 25-34 ☐ 35-44 ☐ 45-54 ☐ 55-64 ☐ 65+

5. **Highest level of education completed?**

   ☐ Did not attend school
   ☐ Some high school
   ☐ Graduated from high school
   ☐ Some college
   ☐ Graduated from college
   ☐ Some graduate school
   ☐ Completed graduate school

6. **Marital Status**

   ☐ Single ☐ Married

7. **Have you ever received diabetes education?**

☐ Yes   ☐ No

8. **Which of the following categories best describes your employment status?**

☐ Employed, working full-time
☐ Employed, working part-time
☐ Not employed
☐ Retired
☐ Disabled, not able to work

APPENDIX D

Diabetes Knowledge Test

Michigan Diabetes Research and Training Center's Revised Diabetes Knowledge Scale

1. **The diabetes diet is:**
   a. the way most American people eat
   b. a healthy diet for most people
   c. too high in carbohydrate for most people
   d. too high in protein for 0 most people

2. **Which of the following is highest in carbohydrate?**
   a. Baked chicken
   b. Swiss cheese
   c. 1 Baked potato
   d. Peanut butter

3. **Which of the following is highest in fat?**
   a. Low fat (2%) milk
   b. Orange juice
   c. Corn
   d. Honey

4. **Which of the 2 following is a "free food"?**
   a. Any unsweetened food
   b. Any food that has "fat free" on the label
   c. Any food that has "sugar free" on the label
   d. Any food that has less than 20 calories per serving

5. **A1C is a measure of your average blood glucose level for the 4 past:**
   a. day
   b. week
   c. 6-12 weeks
   d. 6 months

6. **Which is the best method for home glucose testing?**
   a. Urine testing
   b. Blood testing
   c. Both are equally good

7. **What effect does unsweetened fruit juice have on blood glucose?**

a. Lowers it
b. Raises it
c. Has no effect

8. **Which should <u>not</u> be used to treat low blood glucose?**

a. 3 hard candies
b. 1/2 cup orange juice
c. 1 cup diet soft drink
d. 1 cup skim milk

9. **For a person in good control, what effect does exercise have on blood glucose?**

a. Lowers it
b. Raises it
c. Has no effect

10. **What effect will an infection most likely have on blood glucose?**

a. Lowers it
b. Raises it
c. Has no effect

11. **The best way to take care of your feet is to:**

a. look at and wash them each day
b. massage them with alcohol each day
c. soak them for one hour each day
d. buy shoes a size larger than usual

12. **Eating foods lower in fat decreases your risk for:**

a. nerve disease
b. kidney disease
c. heart disease
d. eye disease

13. **Numbness and tingling may be symptoms of:**

a. nerve disease
b. kidney disease
c. eye disease
d. liver disease

14. **Which of the following is usually not associated with diabetes:**

a. vision problems
b. kidney problems
c. nerve problems
d. lung problems

15. **Signs of ketoacidosis (DKA) include:**

a. shakiness
b. sweating
c. vomiting
d. low blood glucose

16. **If you are sick with the flu, you should:**

a. Take less insulin
b. Drink less liquids
c. Eat more proteins
d. Test blood glucose more often

17. **If you have taken rapid-acting insulin, you are most likely to have a low blood glucose reaction in:**
    a. Less than 2 hours
    b. 3-5 hours
    c. 6-12 hours
    d. More than 13 hours

18. **You realize just before lunch that you forgot to take your insulin at breakfast. What should you do now?**
    a. Skip lunch to lower your blood glucose
    b. Take the insulin that you usually take at breakfast
    c. Take twice as much insulin as you usually take at breakfast
    d. Check your blood glucose level to decide how much insulin to take

19. **If you are beginning to have a low blood glucose reaction, you should:**
    a. exercise
    b. lie down and rest
    c. drink some juice
    d. take rapid-acting insulin

20. **A low blood glucose reaction may be caused by:**
    a. too much insulin
    b. too little insulin
    c. too much food
    d. too little exercise

21. **If you take your morning insulin but skip breakfast, your blood glucose level will usually:**
    a. increase
    b. decrease
    c. remain the same

22. **High blood glucose may be caused by:**
    a. not enough insulin
    b. skipping meals
    c. delaying your snack
    d. skipping your exercise

23. **A low blood glucose reaction may be caused by:**
    a. heavy exercise
    b. infection
    c. overeating
    d. not taking your insulin

Scoring

Correct answers for the DKT

1 = b	8 = c	15 = c
2 = c	9 = a	16 = d
3 = a	10 = b	17 = a
4 = d	11 = a	18 = d
5 = c	12 = c	19 = c
6 = b	13 = b	20 = b
7 = b	14 = d	21 = b

APPENDIX E

The Summary of Diabetes Self-Care Activities Scale

The questions below ask you about your diabetes self-care activities during the past 7 days. If you were sick during the past 7 days, please think back to the last 7 days that you were not sick.

Diet		Number of days							
		0	1	2	3	4	5	6	7
1	On how many of the last SEVEN DAYS have you follo your eating plan?								
2	On Average, over the past month, how many DAYS PER WEEK have you followed your eating plan?								
3	On how many of the last SEVEN DAYS did you eat five or more servings of fruits and vegetables?								
4	On how many of the last SEVEN DAYS did you eat high fat foods such as red meat or full-fat dairy products?								
5	On how many of the last SEVEN DAYS did you space carbohydrates evenly through the day?								

Physical Activity and Exercise		Number of days							
		0	1	2	3	4	5	6	7
6	On how many of the last SEVEN DAYS did you participate in at least 30 minutes of physical activity? (Total minutes of continuous activity, including walking).								
7	On how many of the last SEVEN DAYS did you participate in a specific exercise session (such as such swimming, walking, biking) other than what you do around the house or as part of your work?								

Blood Sugar Testing		Number of days							
		0	1	2	3	4	5	6	7
8	On how many of the last SEVEN DAYS did you participate in at least 30 minutes of physical activity? *(Total minutes of continuous activity, including walking).*								
9	On how many of the last SEVEN DAYS did you participate in a specific exercise session (such as such swimming, walking, biking) other than what you do around the house or as part of your work?								

Foot Care		Number of days							
		0	1	2	3	4	5	6	7
10	On how many of the last SEVEN DAYS did you check your feet?								
11	On how many of the last SEVEN DAYS did you inspect the inside of your shoes?								
12	On how many of the last SEVEN DAYS did you wash your feet?								
13	On how many of the last SEVEN DAYS did you soak your feet?								
14	On how many of the last SEVEN DAYS did you dry between your toes after washing?								

Medication		Number of days							
		0	1	2	3	4	5	6	7
15	On how many of the last SEVEN DAYS did you take your recommended diabetes medication?								

Scoring

Scoring Instructions for the Summary of Diabetes Self-Care Activities

(Expanded)

Scores are calculated for each of the five regimen areas assessed by the SDSCA: Diet, Exercise, Blood-Glucose Testing, Foot Care, and Medication.

Step 1

For items 1–15, use the number of days per week on a scale of 0–7. Note that this response scale will not allow for direct comparison with the percentages provided in Table 1.

Step 2: Scoring Scales

General Diet = Mean number of days for items 1 and 2.

Specific Diet = Mean number of days for items 3, 4 and 5, reversing item 4 (0=7, 1=6, 2=5, 3=4, 4=3, 5=2, 6=1, 7=0). Given the low inter-item correlations for this scale, using the individual items is recommended.

Exercise = Mean number of days for items 6 and 7.

Blood-Glucose Testing = Mean number of days for items 8 and 9.

Foot Care = Mean number of days for items 10 to 14, after reversing 13 (0=7, 1=6, 2=5, 3=4, 4=3, 5=2, 6=1, 7=0).

Medications = Use total number of days for item 15.

APPENDIX F

Stanford Diabetes Self-care efficacy Scale

We would like to know how confident you are in doing certain activities. For each of the following questions, please circle the number that corresponds to your confidence that you can do the tasks regularly at the present time.

1.) How confident do you feel that you can eat your meals every 4 to 5 hours every day, including breakfast every day?

not at all confident   totally confident

1   2   3   4   5   6   7   8   9   10

2.) How confident do you feel that you can follow your diet when you have to prepare or share foodwith other people who do nothave diabetes?

not at all confident   totally confident

1   2   3   4   5   6   7   8   9   10

3.) How confident do you feel that you can choose the appropriate foods to eat when you are hungry (for example, snacks)?

not at all confident   totally confident

1   2   3   4   5   6   7   8   9   10

4.) How confident do you feel that you can exercise 15 to 30 minutes, 4 to 5 times a week?

not at all confident   totally confident

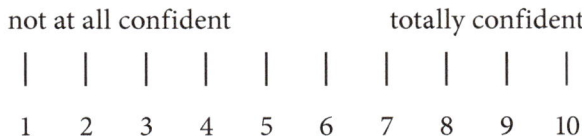

1   2   3   4   5   6   7   8   9   10

5.) How confident do you feel that you can do something to prevent your blood sugar level from dropping when you exercise

not at all confident   totally confident

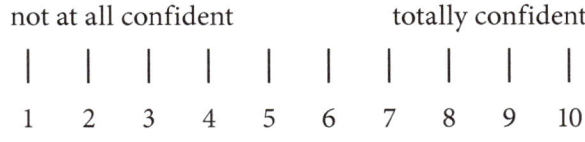
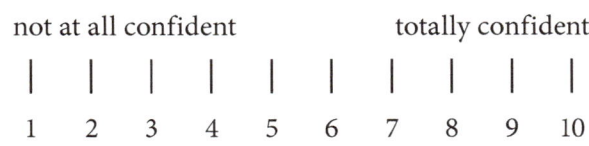

1   2   3   4   5   6   7   8   9   10

6.) How confident do you feel that you know what to do when your blood sugar level goes higher or lower than it should be?

not at all confident   totally confident

| 1 | 2 | 3 | 4 | 5 | 6 | 7 | 8 | 9 | 10 |

7.) How confident do you feel that you can judge when the changes in your illness mean you should visit the doctor?

not at all confident   totally confident

| 1 | 2 | 3 | 4 | 5 | 6 | 7 | 8 | 9 | 10 |

8.) How confident do you feel that you can control your diabetes so that it does not interfere with the things you want to do?

not at all confident   totally confident

| 1 | 2 | 3 | 4 | 5 | 6 | 7 | 8 | 9 | 10 |

Scoring

The score for each item is the number circled. If two consecutive numbers are circled, code the lower number (less self-care efficacy). If the numbers are not consecutive, do not score the item. The score for the scale is the mean of the eight items. If more than two items are missing, do not score the scale. Higher number indicates higher self-care efficacy.

Characteristics

Test on 86 subjects with diabetes.

No. of Observed	Standard Internal Consistency	Test-Retest items	Range Mean	Deviation Reliability	Reliability
8	1-10	6.87	1.76	8.28	NA

Source of Psychometric Data

Stanford English Diabetes Self-Management study. Study reported in Lorig K, Ritter PL, Villa FJ, Armas J. Community-Based Peer-Led Diabetes Self-Management: A Randomized Trial. The Diabetes Educator 2009; Jul-Aug; 35(4):641-51.

Comments

This 8-item scale was originally developed and tested in Spanish for the Diabetes Self-Management study. For internet studies, we add radio buttons below each number. There is another way that we use to format these items, which takes up less space on a questionnaire, shown also in the PDF document. This scale is available in Spanish.

This scale is free to use without permission

Self-Management Resource Center
711 Colorado Avenue Palo Alto CA 94303
(650) 242-8040 smrc@selfmanagementresource.com
www.selfmanagementresource.com

APPENDIX G

Results of Binary Logistics Regression Model

Table 17. Contribution of variables to the model

Omnibus Tests of Model Coefficients				
		Chi-square	df	Sig.
Step 1	Step	136.971	7	.000
	Block	136.971	7	.000
	Model	136.971	7	.000

Model Summary			
		Cox & Snell R	
Step	-2 Log likelihood	Square	Nagelkerke R Square
1	27.747[a]	.681	.912
a. Estimation terminated at iteration number 11 because parameter estimates changed by less than .001			

Hosmer and Lemeshow Test			
Step	Chi-square	df	Sig.
1	2.992	8	.935

Classification Table[a]

	Observed		Predicted		
			Diabetes education		Percentage Correct
			No	Yes	
Step 1	Diabetes education	No	64	3	95.5
		Yes	2	51	96.2
	Overall Percentage				95.8

a. The cut value is .500

Variables in the Equation

		B	S.E.	Wald	df	Sig.	Exp(B)
Step 1[a]	Combined knowledge score (1 - 23)	.444	.312	2.024	1	.155	1.559
	Combined Self-care Management	1.082	.415	6.786	1	.009	2.951
	Combined Self-care Efficacy	-.076	.079	.916	1	.339	.927
	Medication type	-1.239	.881	1.979	1	.159	.290
	Duration of illness	1.799	1.162	2.396	1	.122	6.043
	Age group	-2.016	1.627	1.535	1	.215	.133
	Level of education	.319	.565	.318	1	.573	1.375
	Constant	-98.685	36.689	7.235	1	.007	.000

a. Variable(s) entered on step 1: Combined knowledge score (1 - 23), Combined Self-care Management, Combined Self-care Efficacy, Medication type, Duration of illness, Age group, Level of education.